THE THERAPEUTIC
RELATIONSHIP
IN BEHAVIOURAL
PSYCHOTHERAPY

WILEY SERIES IN
PSYCHOTHERAPY AND COUNSELLING

SERIES EDITORS
Franz Epting, *Dept of Psychology, University of Florida, USA*
Bonnie Strickland, *Dept of Psychology, University of Massachusetts, USA*
John Allen, *Dept of Community Studies, University of Brighton, UK*

Self, Symptoms and Psychotherapy
Edited by Neil Cheshire and Helmut Thomae

Beyond Sexual Abuse: Therapy with Women who were Childhood Victims
Derek Jehu

Cognitive-Analytic Therapy: Active Participation in Change: A New Integration in Brief Psychotherapy
Anthony Ryle

The Power of Countertransference: Innovations in Analytic Technique
Karen J. Maroda

Strategic Family Play Therapy
Shlomo Ariel

The Evolving Professional Self: Stages and Themes in Therapist and Counselor Development
Thomas M. Skovholt and Michael Helge Rønnestad

Feminist Perspectives in Therapy: An Empowerment Model for Women
Judith Worell and Pam Remer

Counselling and Therapy with Refugees: Psychological Problems of Victims of War, Torture and Repression
Guus van der Veer

Psychoanalytic Counseling
Michael J. Patton and Naomi M. Meara

Life Stories: Personal Construct Therapy with the Elderly
Linda L. Viney

Being and Belonging: Group, Intergruop and Gestalt
Gaie Houston

The Therapeutic Relationship in Behavioural Psychotherapy
Cas Schaap, Ian Bennun, Ludwig Schindler and Kees Hoogduin

Further titles in preparation

THE THERAPEUTIC RELATIONSHIP IN BEHAVIOURAL PSYCHOTHERAPY

Cas Schaap

Ian Bennun

Ludwig Schindler *and*

Kees Hoogduin

John Wiley & Sons
Chichester • New York • Brisbane • Toronto • Singapore

Other Wiley Editorial Offices

John Wiley & Sons, Inc., 605 Third Avenue,
New York, NY 10158-0012, USA

Jacaranda Wiley Ltd, G.P.O. Box 859, Brisbane,
Queensland 4001, Australia

John Wiley & Sons (Canada) Ltd, 22 Worcester Road,
Rexdale, Ontario M9W 1L1, Canada

John Wiley & Sons (SEA) Pte Ltd, 37 Jalan Pemimpin #05-04,
Block B, Union Industrial Building, Singapore 2057

Library of Congress Cataloging-in-Publication Data

The therapeutic relationship in behavioural psychotherapy / Cas Schaap
... [et al.].
    p.   cm.
  Includes bibliographical references and index.
  ISBN 0-471-92458-X
  1. Behavior therapy.   2. Psychotherapist and patient.   I. Schaap,
Cas, *1945–*   .
  [DNLM: 1. Psychotherapy.   2. Behaviour therapy.   3. Professional
–Patient Relations.   WM 425 T3983 1993]
RC489.B4T545   1993
616.89'142—dc20
DNLM/DLC
for Library of Congress   93–16587
                                                                        CIP

British Library Cataloguing in Publication Data

A catalogue record for this book is available from the British Library

ISBN 0-471-92458-X

Typeset in 10/12pt Times from authors' disks by Text Processing Department,
John Wiley & Sons Ltd, Chichester
Printed and bound in Great Britain by Biddles, Guildford, Surrey

Contents

Series Preface

TheWiley Series in Psychotherapy and Counseling is designed to fulfil many different needs in advancing knowledge and practice in the helping professions. What unifies the books in this series is the importance attached to presenting clear authorative accounts of theory, research and experience in ways which will inform practice and understanding.

The Therapeutic Relationship in Behavioural Psychotherapy is an important book. For too long behavioural psychotherapy has been seen as a collection of techniques devoid of any real concern with the relationship between therapist and client. The authors of the present volume argue that while that description may well have applied to earlier behavioural approaches such a view is no longer tenable. Indeed as a description of effective behavioural psychotherapy it has always been seriously misleading. Here, for the first time, is a comprehensive integration of research on the therapeutic relationshipand the principles of behavioural psychotherapy. By means of a thorough review of research on common and specific factors over a wide range of therapeutic approaches, the authors show how an integrative model of behavioural psychotherapy can be established.

The process model of behavioural psychotherapy developed in this volume is likely to have aprofound influence on future generations of therapists. It provides a way of understanding the changes in the therapeuticrealtionship over the course of therapy, and integrates insights from social influence research and behavioural/cognitive therapy. The authors also offer a model of managing the therapeutic relationship which is based upon both research and extensive clinical practice.

Many counsellors and psychotherapists who have felt attracted to the rigour and rationality of behavioural approaches have been deterred by the absence of any real consideration of the therapeutic relationship. This volume fills that gap and will, no doubt, revitalize interest in, and enthusiasm for, behavioural psychotherapy.

It is with great pleasure that this volume is welcomed to the series.

John Allen
Series Editor

Preface

The therapeutic relationship is a recent discovery in behavioural psychotherapy. Where other psychotherapy schools have, in their own specific ways, emphasized a good working relationship and a therapeutic relationship of high quality, behaviour therapists have focused instead, on the effectiveness of treatment techniques, particularly in their empirical research. In doing so, they have neglected the fact that treatment techniques are delivered in a social setting: the therapeutic setting. It is the aim of this book to point out the importance of the therapeutic relationship for effective implementation of techniques. Our position is rooted in the convictions that (a) the relationship between client and therapist is the most important common factor in any healing situation, and (b) this relationship can be managed.

The book is divided into three parts. In the first part we describe the importance of common and nonspecific factors in psychotherapy. The impact of common factors—factors that are considered to be common to the different healing practices—and non specific factors—factors operative in the healing practice that are not considered to be an essential ingredient of that treatment in the theoretical view of the healer—has been established in different fields of research, and has been shown in the comparison of different schools of psychotherapy.

We then point out the position of the different psychotherapeutic schools with regard to the importance of the therapeutic relationship and the outcome of research into common factors. Studies show that behaviour therapy has a characteristic style, which is different from other schools. Though it is somewhat surprising, behaviour therapists have been rated higher on relationship variables such as empathy, unconditional positive regard and congruence than have Gestalt therapists and psychodynamic psychotherapists. These results clearly contradict the traditional stereotype of the cold and mechanistic behaviour therapist.

We end Part 1 by describing a process model of behavioural psychotherapy comprised of seven phases that constitutes a bridge between assumptions of social influence, developed within the field of social psychology, and the structuring of the therapy process that is typical for behavioural psychotherapy. Therapy is considered a co-operative process of problem solving to which explicitly interpersonal aspects are added. Although the different phases are often difficult to distinguish in reality, they represent an attempt at conceptualizing the progress of the therapeutic influence from the inception of the therapeutic relationship, over the application of techniques of intervention, towards the dissolution of the therapeutic bond.

In the second part of this volume a model of managing the therapeutic relationship is described, derived from clinical practice. This model is based on an extensive literature survey of specific strategies to influence clients, ranging from popular books on salesmanship to (client-centred and interpersonal) literature on dealing with problematic clients. In these three chapters we challenge the long-cherished proposition that clients must adapt to the therapists' psychotherapeutic style in order for behaviour change to occur. Change is most likely to occur if therapists adapt to the way clients view their role in the change process and present themselves. We demonstrate how therapists can change their behaviour in ways that enable clients to experience the relationship more positively, to participate actively, and thus succeed in the treatment goals.

In Part 3 we present a review of process research and of instruments measuring aspects of the quality of the therapeutic relationship. We expand further the methodological aspects of a systematic assessment and outline the important instruments that are used to assess the different aspects of the therapeutic relationship. In order to gain more empirical knowledge about strategies of social influence and their impact within the therapeutic interaction, we present the outcome of research on the actual process of change within and across therapy sessions. The final chapter focuses on the findings of studies that have used these procedures. More specifically, research is presented that examines the relationship between behavioural style and treatment outcome, and on studies using behavioural observational measures. The book ends with an integrative conclusion and recommendations for future research.

Part 1
THEORETICAL
FOUNDATIONS

In Chapter 1 the importance of the relationship between therapist and patient is described for the different schools of psychotherapy, including behavioural psychotherapy. The therapeutic relationship might well be termed *the* common factor in treatment. In Chapter 2 a process-oriented model of therapeutic change is presented.

1 The therapeutic relationship: the common factor in psychotherapy

Introduction: common and nonspecific factors in healing

Since the pioneering work of Jerome Frank (1973), an increased interest among psychotherapists and researchers in common and nonspecific factors in healing has been evident. The impact of *common* factors, that is, factors that are considered to be common to the different healing practices, and of *nonspecific* factors, those factors operative in the healing practice that are not considered in the healer's theoretical view to be an essential ingredient of a specific treatment, has been established in different fields of research and psychotherapy (Garfield, 1981; Shapiro & Shapiro, 1982; Smith, Glass & Miller, 1980).

Though the validity of the conclusion that the different schools of psychotherapy are equally effective is often questioned (Prioleau, Murdock & Brody, 1983), the importance of the nonspecific and common factors in the various established schools of Western psychotherapies is less questionable (Frank, 1973). In various studies of psychotherapy it is reported that about 65% of clients treated improve. There are, however, a number of methodological problems that must be taken into account when interpreting this figure:

1 The difficulties in accurately assessing complaints, which in turn influence the dependent variables in outcome studies.
2 The sometimes tenuous relationship between the treatment and its effect; the so-called integrity of treatment.
3 The implementation of the treatment and its effect.
4 The implementation of the design.

The nonspecific and common factors have their impact in any healing situation, not only psychotherapy but also alternative methods.

4 Theoretical foundations

Improvement rates in the treatment of a wide range of conditions using alternative healing methods, such as acupuncture, magnetism and other paranormal methods, are quite impressive; these rates are in many ways comparable to those of the established forms of Western psychotherapy, which may be suggestive of the importance of common or nonspecific factors (Krippner, 1975; Vahia, 1973; Van Dijk, 1979; Van Kalmthout, Schaap & Wojciechowski, 1985).

Van Dijk (1979) reported an overall success rate of 90% achieved by Chinese acupuncturists, and a rate of 84% of cases treated by acupuncturists in the former Soviet Union and China. About the same improvement rate is reported for established schools of psychotherapy, if improvement for neurotic and psychosomatic conditions is calculated (Van Dijk, 1979). The same figure was reported by Gouwe (1961) for the effectiveness of paranormal methods and by Vahia (1973) for yoga. Although one might doubt the reliability of these figures, there is little doubt about the presence of important nonspecific or common factors within these alternative healing practices.

Non-Western healing practices are also in many ways comparable to the different forms of Western psychotherapies, both in process as well as outcome (Jilek, 1974; Nawas, Pluk & Wojciechowski, 1985; Prince, 1964; Torrey, 1972). Prince (1964) observed 50 witch doctors of the Yoruba tribe in Nigeria and concluded that they were as effective as Western psychiatrists. Jilek (1974) spent 6 years studying the Coast Salish Indian tribes in British Columbia, and concluded that their improvement rates were certainly not inferior to those reported by Western healers. Similar results were reported by Torrey (1972) on the basis of his observations of witch doctors in such varying regions of the world as Ethiopia, Serawak, Bali, Hong Kong and different subcultures in the U.S.A. The fact that these figures are comparable with those reported for treatments by paraprofessionals (Durlak, 1979; Hattie, Sharpley & Rogers, 1984; Strupp, 1978) is further proof of the impact of theoretically unspecified, yet common, factors in a variety of healing settings in research on psychotherapy outcome, particularly if it is controlled for credibility of the rationale, and suggests that the same processes are at work under these conditions (Nawas et al, 1985; Prioleau et al, 1983; Rosenthal, 1980; Shapiro, 1986; Wilson & Evans, 1977). A crucial ingredient of these procedures is the establishment of an intense relationship, characterized by such complementary features as trustworthiness, dependency, emotional arousal, directness, disclosure and responsivity (Frank, 1973; Nawas et al, 1985; Pope, 1979).

Jerome Frank (1973) was one of the first authors to point out that contemporary scientific principles of Western psychotherapy, as well as the so-called primitive and alternative healing practices, share many structural and procedural similarities. He assumed that these common factors form the important ingredients in effective psychotherapy. Cultural factors are important to the extent that they determine the value of a theoretical explanation and the content of the healing procedures. According to Frank, one may claim that psychotherapy aims to alleviate psychological suffering and, as such, focuses on a fundamental change in the patient's cognitions, emotions and behaviour. Psychotherapy tries to relieve the patients' complaints, while at the same time attempts to change patients to such an extent that they will be able to function more effectively. These two goals of psychotherapy, *symptom reduction* and a fundamental *personal change*, are based on two different processes.

According to Frank, *symptom reduction* is a consequence of the client's expectations regarding the cure for the complaint. He bases this assumption on the observation that reduction in complaints is usually effected relatively early in treatment, regardless of the type of therapy; even in placebo treatments, clients report improvement in well-being despite no treatment taking place.

Mobilizing patients' expectations is only one aspect of therapeutic effectiveness. The reduction in complaints that occurs in placebo treatments, should be viewed mainly as the result of developing and strengthening clients' expectations, whereas the attitude change and the improved self-efficacy are mainly determined by the prestige and status of the therapist, and the specific influence of the techniques that are used.

Client complaints are in part determined by cultural and social factors, and can in part be attributed to a condition of *demoralization*, a state in which clients have lost self-esteem. As a result of losing self-esteem, clients may not feel capable of dealing with further aspects of their lives and in addition may experience feelings of shame and guilt. In such a state, a client runs the risk of becoming socially isolated. From this model, symptoms may be perceived as an expression of this demoralization, as well as a sign of combating these feelings. It is the task of psychotherapy, and indeed of the therapist, to redress this loss of morale. This can be achieved by alleviating the destructive feelings and attitudes, and by stimulating self-confidence, self-control and personal effectiveness. This conviction, which Frank called *sense of mastery*, is indeed the main goal of treatment, and can be described as the sense of having control over the internal resources and the relevant external circumstances.

The way a sense of mastery can be achieved depends on a number of factors, such as experiences of success. Assignments that lead to success will therefore have to be experienced as somewhat difficult, so that they can be labelled as a success. The type of experiences that lead to this increased sense of self-control are therefore mostly determined by the extent to which the clients attribute the success to themselves, that is, their *internal attribution orientation*.

Frank considers psychotherapy to be a special form of social influence. This implies two reciprocal roles: a persuader and a subject. Therapists have to persuade their clients that their rationale for the problem and treatment is valid and that the particular treatment is consequently of importance. In exchange for submission to the therapeutic system and its role relationship, the client receives warmth, support, a way of reducing guilt without losing face and faith in a cure. However, the fact that experiences are being looked at in a different light, that the patient is given the opportunity to confess faults and mistakes in a supportive atmosphere without having to lose face, strengthens the therapeutic relationship. This again reduces anxiety, increases hope and expectation and will, as a consequence, increase the probability of success.

If the above conditions are met, they can only be achieved through an atmosphere that is characterized by high *emotional arousal*. It is this arousal that will enable the client to be more receptive to the influence of the therapist in changing his or her attitudes and behaviour. Different cultures have developed their own ways of achieving this emotional arousal: some of these include rhythmic movements, dramatic performance, catharsis, flooding, sensory deprivation, meditation, hypnosis, relaxation and social isolation. During psychotherapeutic treatment, old values and norms lose their grip, new values and norms have not yet been substituted. This transition is likely to bring the client into an even more emotionally unstable condition. In addition, self-disclosure about the past may result in experiencing negative emotions. Emotional arousal as such, however, is not sufficient to achieve an attitude change. A re-interpretation and restructuring of the client's way of life must also occur, which will need to be consolidated with the support from the social environment.

Cognitive "indoctrination" and the *use of emotional arousal* need to occur within a relationship between patient and healer in order to bring about change. The *therapeutic relationship* is the third important factor in a situation of social influence, that psychotherapy undeniably constitutes. To the patient, the therapist is the most important source of healing. The influence of the therapist increases with the severity of the psychological problems, and as the patient's trust in the skills of the therapist increases. The way clients perceive their therapist depends on their own situation, their personality characteristics and the personal qualities of the therapist, who has a socially sanctioned role with high status. The identity and the status of the therapist as a healer is emphasized by his or her setting and attributes.

Van Dyck (1986) presented an illuminating review of the literature on the effective ingredients of psychotherapy. He begins by questioning whether psychotherapy can be considered as being comparable with placebo treatment, i.e. any treatment where the elements and characteristics of the healing theory are not the therapeutically active ingredients. Placebo effects play a role in physical conditions as well as in psychological disorders. Each new development in treatment approaches helps alter the belief in, and effectiveness of, old treatment methods. The value that a therapist places on the therapy or drug treatment also influences its effectiveness to a considerable degree. The effect of placebo treatments are to a lesser extent affected by personality factors than by the therapists' attitudes and the context of therapy. According to Van Dyck (1986), placebo or nonspecific therapeutic factors lead to a reduction in anxiety and a more positive patient attitude through a commitment to the treatment and expectation about healing.

Van Dyck (1986) showed that specific psychotherapeutic conditions are more effective than placebo conditions and that the latter yield better results than no-treatment control groups (see also Barker, Funk & Houston, 1988). In particular this last finding is further evidence for the fact that next to technical aspects of treatment, relationship factors can lead to change. A constructive relationship between client and therapist seems therefore the condition *sine qua non* for therapeutic change. In order to increase the effectiveness of psychotherapy, these neglected mechanisms of change should be theoretically specified and systematically studied.

Van Dyck (1986) developed an interesting model based on the findings of placebo treatments and the ideas of Jerome Frank. Figure 1.1 indicates the way that the common or placebo elements of therapy lead to the main goal of treatment, that is a sense of mastery and symptom reduction.

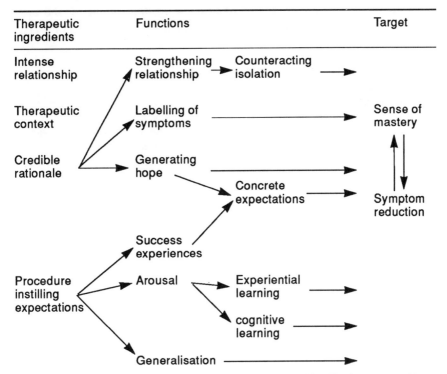

Figure 1.1   Survey of the therapeutic factors (based on Van Dyck, 1986, p.19)

8 Theoretical foundations

No single theory can explain all human problems, and no single therapy can heal them all. The therapist and client do, however, need a common framework to interpret presenting problems. Each psychotherapeutic approach uses, to varying degrees, a theoretical model. How explicit this theory is remains variable and therapists often do not realize that what they do and what they say they do actually differ (Van Dyck & Emmelkamp, 1985). This then necessitates the study of the effective factors in psychotherapy, and the therapeutic relationship, which is likely to increase the effectiveness of common factors. Van Dyck's answer to his question about the comparability of psychotherapy and placebo is that placebo control groups are less effective than many active psychotherapies; however, almost no specific psychotherapy techniques can be identified that are demonstrably more effective than a credible placebo.

In the following sections, we will focus on the most common elements in treatment: the therapeutic relationship and the role of client and therapist as formulated within psychoanalysis, client-centred psychotherapy and behaviour therapy. For each approach, we will describe the historical roots, the theoretical premises, and the value that is placed on the quality of the therapeutic relationship, as well as the research in the area of this relationship. We will go on to review the literature specifically addressing how each theory views client–therapist interaction. This will provide the foundation for the next chapter, which describes a social psychological model of psychotherapy.

The therapeutic relationship in psychoanalysis

Historical aspects

Although we are well aware of the variation in and developments of the theory and practice of psychoanalysis (e.g. Davanloo, 1978; Luborsky, 1984), we will focus here on traditional psychoanalytic therapy. According to psychoanalytic theory, neuroses are cured by exploring certain aspects of past life and discovering their causal connections to present life. The basic assumption is that current symptoms originate from unconscious conflicts. The therapeutic process consists primarily of allowing these conflicts to surface to consciousness. A neurotic conflict is solved when those parts of the Ego, the Id and Superego are integrated after having been rejected from consciousness during natural growth. The purpose of treatment is to motivate the Ego to relinquish pathological defence mechanisms or to find more appropriate ones. These structural changes in the Ego are considered as the only viable solution to the basic conflicts and are, by the same token, the guarantee for permanent change.

The central therapeutic technique, which allows for relevant information to be available for this process, is *free association*. This technique is based on

Freud's assumption that unconscious content strives towards expression by trying to cross the frontiers of the Ego and become conscious. As a ground rule, clients are encouraged to say anything that comes to mind, even when the content seems illogical or is experienced as unpleasant. With the assistance of the therapist, this material is then analysed through insight-oriented techniques, such as confrontation, clarification, interpretation and working through.

Theoretical aspects

Within psychoanalysis the relationship between client and therapist is of the utmost importance. The psychoanalytic process may therefore be described as an interaction between client and therapist that results in structural changes within the client's psychological make-up. A working alliance has to be established between therapist and client which is relatively non-neurotic and rational. This relationship then enables the patient to work in a goal-directed way in the analytic situation and implies the capability of working analytically with the new insights. The analyst contributes to the process by applying a particular therapeutic style that is characterized by understanding and insight, as well as an empathic, honest and nonevaluative attitude. This analytical atmosphere is seen as the condition for the patient to accept the interpretations.

Throughout treatment, the therapeutic relationship itself becomes the object of analysis. It is assumed that neurotic patients tend to show transference reactions in which the client seeks unconscious objects—in this case the therapist—towards which libidinal and aggressive drives are directed. This means that patients tend to relive the past relationships within the treatment in an effort to seek gratification. Such repetitions can lead towards strong libidinal, dependent or aggressive behaviour patterns towards the therapist.

Transference reactions are of great importance and are stimulated by the therapist, since they constitute the essential material of the analysis. Transference reactions may be positive or negative; the former includes such reactions as sympathy, love and respect for the therapist and provides a foundation for the working alliance and leads the patient to identifying with the attitude and method of the analyst. The patient is further helped by perceiving situations differently and trying out new ways of functioning. In negative transference reactions, the patient acts out old conflicts. If the transference reaction becomes a form of resistance, it then has to become the object of the analysis. All unconscious forces that hinder the process of analytic work, are labelled as resistance. Resistance occurs in varying degree throughout the course of treatment and consists of more than just the transference phenomena. Resistance is a defence against the status quo of neurosis and may be considered as a struggle to not relinquish a way of living, however frustrating, if no better alternatives are available. The analysis of this resistance is considered an important analytic task, since it constitutes repeated use of defence mechanisms.

Unconscious affective reactions from the therapist towards the patient are described as counter-transference. A positive attitude of the therapist towards the patient seems to be a necessary condition for a successful course of analysis. However, if this attitude crosses a certain critical point, it can move the patient towards the gratification of a dependency need. It then becomes a hindrance in treatment and may even become ethically questionable. Positive and negative counter-transference become the personal challenge for analysts in their personal growth.

This short description of orthodox psychoanalysis demonstrates that the therapeutic relationship is considered to be at least as important as the techniques of analysis. Factors that are emphasized in psychoanalysis and may be viewed as common factors are the following:

1   Emphasis on the working alliance.
2   The alliance between the client and therapist.
3   A goal-directed course of treatment.
4   An empathic, nondirective, and nonevaluative style of treatment.
5   The client's identification with the therapist.
6   The acceptance of insights and the analytic methods.

Although a number of developments have changed in the practice of psychoanalysis, the therapeutic relationship remains a crucial factor of importance.

Empirical findings

Empirical studies of the therapeutic process in psychoanalysis strengthen notions of the importance of the therapeutic relationship. It appears that the personality characteristics of the therapist and the patient explain only a small amount of variance in therapeutic success (Luborsky, 1976). In contrast, the specific interaction within the therapeutic dyad shows a significant relationship with outcome. If a good working alliance is established in the early stage of treatment, a positive outcome can be predicted (Hartley & Strupp, 1982). In order to a develop a working relationship, more than client motivation is required. Lack of empathy, interest and sensitivity, as well as destructive tendencies on the part of the therapist, can hinder a positive course of treatment (Singer & Luborsky, 1977). Four aspects of the therapist's behaviour are important in establishing a constructive working relationship: (1) directive behaviour, (2) an assertive demeanour, (3) warmth and care, and (4) sensitivity. Some of these elements we will again encounter in the research on therapeutic factors in both client-centred and behaviour therapy.

The therapeutic relationship in client-centred therapy

Historical aspects

Client-centred therapy is based on a personality model emphasizing continuous growth or *self-actualization*. The ideal goal of actualization is a completely developed personality and the tendency to move into the direction of maturity. This development occurs as a result of personal experiences (self) that can only occur in relationships with others. Many experiences are symbolic, yet they can be made conscious.

Theoretical aspects

Pychological adaptation exists with the establishment of the self-concept. This means that all physical and sensory experiences of the organism are assimilated on a symbolic level, in a relationship that is congruent with the concept of self. Psychological adaptation is required, in the sense that people will increasingly become more self-assured and congruent if in their contacts with other persons, they feel accepted and understood.

In contrast, if a person experiences ignoring or nonacceptance of their own subjective internal world, and even coldness and disregard, then this will affect their psychological functioning. If an individual is continually confronted with this attitude, in, for example their school, work or marriage, then this will result in low self-esteem and a negative self-concept. The self-concept then becomes based completely on evaluations of experiences from others. Since the internalized evaluations of others do not have a necessary relationship with the factual experiential world, they will increasingly be expressed as a feeling of tension and pain.

Experiences that are inconsistent with the structure of the self may be perceived as a threat and will be ignored, disavowed and resisted. If this happens repeatedly, the self-structure becomes inflexible as a way of surviving, resulting in a barrier in the development of the personality. Disintegration and disorganization occur when an important event confronts a person who exists in this incongruent state. The person behaves in a disorganized fashion if his/her behaviour is guided on one occasion by his/her self-concept and on another by the disavowed experiences. The aim of client-centred psychotherapy is to relieve this disorganization and to overcome the resistance. A realistic perception can be re-established that will change the structure of the self and will increase its acceptance.

Since interpersonal relationships are considered to either foster or to hinder the development of the self, the therapy is considered as the offering of a relationship that is structured and that will facilitate the potential for growth. Rogers is assumed to have formulated principles that are considered to render such a relationship as helpful. He describes the following six conditions that are considered necessary and sufficient for changing the personality:

1 Two persons engage in a relationship that is meaningful to both of them.
2 The client is in a condition of incongruence, that is "unwhole", vulnerable and anxious. He/she is involved in experiencing and feelings that do not fit with his/her self-image.
3 The therapist provides a congruent and integrated relationship.
4 The therapist is unconditional and accepts any experiences from the client because they constitute this unique person.
5 The therapist experiences the inner world of the client using empathy. He/she tries to reflect the experiences encountered back to the client.
6 The client should show the willingness to accept, at least in principle, the message from the therapist about how he experienced the client unconditionally and how the client is understood.

The conditions 3 to 5 above, contain the therapeutic characteristics that are described as the Rogerian conditions of *congruence, unconditional positive regard* and *empathy*. The therapeutic relationship is understood as a working alliance in which the therapist has no other goal than to establish a relationship as described above. If clients can accept the offer of an empathic, unconditional and congruent relationship, this will define their behaviour and by the same token the therapist's response. Rogers suggests that therapeutic effectiveness does not lie in the establishment of a successful therapeutic relationship, but in the therapist's continuously active endeavour in maintaining this relationship.

A number of streams in client-centred psychotherapy can be distinguished: (experiential psychotherapy (Gendlin, 1973), the more cognitive approach by Rice (Wexler & Rice, 1974) and the more didactic–structured approach by Truax and Carkhuff (Carkhuff, 1969)). This divergence and diversity can be interpreted as a logical consequence of the Rogerian philosophy to find one's way using a personal, experience-oriented method. These approaches do not differ from the "orthodox" view on the therapeutic relationship. This relationship is, however, given a more central role in the "interpersonal" approach.

Kiesler (1982) formulated the essentials of interpersonal psychotherapy as a more directive and interactionally oriented branch of client-centred or person-oriented psychotherapy. The client–therapist interaction, despite its unique characteristics, is in many ways similar to any other human transaction. In such a relationship, the therapist is a participant and an observer.

Furthermore, the client presents the therapist with the same rigid and evoking messages (Beier, 1966) that are sent to others. The first important task for the therapist is to attend to, identify and assess the client's distinctive evoking style as it unfolds in interactions. A major source of this assessment includes the therapists' own emotional reactions experienced during these transactions, as well as the rules that have been developed and which may be hampering their role in the relationship.

The goal of interpersonal treatment is for the therapist and client to identify, clarify, and establish alternatives for the client's rigid and self-defeating evoking style. Their task is to replace constricted, counter-productive transactions by more flexible and clearer communications that are adaptable to the changing realities of specific encounters. It is important that the therapist does not respond in the same ways as significant others have done previously, but rather, responds antisocially and remains focused on the topics and themes of the treatment and the evolving interaction style.

Empirical findings

Rogers' proposals that the therapeutic conditions of empathy, unconditional positive regard and congruence are necessary and sufficient for therapeutic change remain controversial. Many studies have tried to assess whether these conditions are necessary and/or sufficient, but most of these studies are characterized by methodological weaknesses. All of the scales used to operationalize and measure the therapist and client characteristics are inconsistent with the basic concepts (Frank, 1985). Usually, different segments of one or more therapy sessions are used to describe therapist behaviour. However, this procedure only partly reflects the hypothesized process characteristic of the therapeutic relationship. There are also instances when observers have rated clients' and therapists' behaviour without using discrete behavioural categories. However, in this way, no relationship between different therapist and client behaviours can be shown. If they were used appropriately, then researchers would be able to study the mutual influence of both partners at any moment in the therapeutic process (Rice, 1983).

A number of review articles have critically summarized the empirical findings (Lambert, De Julio & Stein, 1978; Parloff, Waskow & Wolfe, 1978). Parloff et al (1978) conclude that after 20 years of research, the evidence for the Rogerian conditions remains unconvincing. Moreover, therapists themselves have revised the original client-centred postulates. In 1976, 702 members of the German Association for Rogerian Psychotherapy were asked about their method of therapy. Only 9% of the respondents maintained the orthodox Rogerian conditions and one-third of the respondents often included non-Rogerian ingredients. Many therapists report using unorthodox techniques such as role play and relaxation.

Eymael (1986) distinguished between a traditional, "reflective" group and an "interaction-oriented" group on the basis of the results of a log book that therapists kept of each session. The results of the treatments of 26 outpatients showed an interesting pattern; the latter group—by using confrontation, interpretation and discussion of the therapeutic relationship—had better outcome with their clients than the former group. Actually, this latter group of therapists appeared as effective as the behaviour-oriented therapists in that study. This suggests that client-centred therapists in practice have a need for a broader spectrum of intervention techniques and seem more directive. Based on their theoretical foundation, client-centred therapists strongly emphasize the importance of the therapeutic relationship. One could even say, and one would not be underrating other factors in psychotherapeutic practice, that the therapeutic relationship is considered the primary vehicle for therapeutic change.

The therapeutic relationship in behaviour therapy

Historical aspects

Behaviour therapy is the therapeutic school that has been known for emphasizing techniques for which the therapeutic relationship was a relatively neglected aspect and was considered to be a nonspecific factor. Since behaviour therapy originated from a dissatisfaction with the more traditional approaches, this neglect of the therapeutic relationship is understandable. It has instead, endeavoured to focus in research on the structural and technical aspects of the therapy process.

The origins of behaviour therapy are characterized by the attempt to implement the notions of the psychology of learning in the treatment of psychological problems, and to emphasize the experimental character of therapy. The early behaviour therapists saw themselves as laboratory researchers, as trainers and even as behavioural engineers. The intervention technique was the only factor responsible for therapeutic success, and the identity and behaviour of the therapist were considered irrelevant.

In the early publications (i.e. Wolpe, 1958) there are reports that those clients who improved had established a positive relationship with their therapists before the effective techniques had been applied. These observations remained largely ignored by other behaviour therapists and researchers. But therapists of other orientations who have taken a closer look at the practice of behaviour therapy, Locke (1971), for example, showed that Wolpe's clinical work could not be described in behavioural terms alone. Similarly, other authors, for example Patterson (1968), concluded that clinical practice involved more than could be gleaned from scientific publications. Behaviour therapists offer suggestive utterances and develop a personal and empathic style of interaction with their clients.

The resulting controversies remained largely on a philosophical and ideological level, and unfortunately succeeded in effectively blocking the development of systematic and empirical study of the therapeutic relationship. Only after having established itself as a therapeutic school in its own right and having refined its intervention techniques, did this change. Increasingly it became apparent that focusing on just the technical aspects of the therapeutic process implied a self-imposed limitation of the heuristic value of the theoretical model. When it was recognized that behaviour can be influenced by interpersonal factors as well as techniques, then a new arena of experimental research opened up that provided the opportunity for a better understanding of both the therapeutic process and increased efficacy.

Several studies have demonstrated the significance of the therapeutic relationship for both therapists (e.g. Swan & McDonald, 1978) and clients (Llewellyn & Hume, 1979; Ryan & Gyzynsky, 1971; Staples, Sloane, Whipple, Cristol & Yorkson, 1975). Many surveys have appeared in recent years that have focused on the therapeutic relationship, a topic too often ignored in behaviour therapy (DeVoge & Beck, 1978; Rosenthal, 1980; Sweet, 1984; Wilson & Evans, 1976, 1977). The therapeutic relationship is connected with several types of disturbances (e.g. Lenihan & Sanders, 1984). However, it is recognized that further development within behaviour therapy will be limited if therapists continue to ignore the need to integrate a more comprehensive theory of human relationships within their model (DeVoge & Beck, 1978).

Theoretical aspects

During the early development of behaviour therapy, it was assumed that if a client discussed anxiety-provoking themes with a warm and empathic therapist, a process of desensitization would occur. If the therapist was not punitive then the anxiety would be reduced, an assumption first reported by Dollard and Miller (1950) and later again taken up by Martin (1971), who was trying to integrate behaviour therapy with client-centred therapy. This notion seems interesting from the point of view of an explanation of the efficacy of the variables in treatment. However, it is not a sufficient explanation of other events that occur within behaviour therapy. Moreover, these ideas about a desensitization effect of the therapeutic relationship have remained present in theoretical discussions but have not resulted in further empirical explanations.

Within the operant paradigm, the behavioural engineers of the 1960s attempted to create the conditions for change by establishing contingencies in the therapy sessions. This approach culminated in Krasner's (1962) publication, describing the therapist as a "social reinforcement machine". These ideas were based on the result of the experiments on verbal conditioning which had shown that the occurrence of particular classes of words could be influenced by conditioning. From our present-day perspective, it is considered doubtful that social reinforcement automatically increases a response.

Several studies have indicated that the effects of verbal conditioning are more pronounced when subjects know the purpose and the problem. The conditioning effect is apparently determined by the person's awareness, motivation and skill in formulating hypotheses about the target class (Spielberger & DeNike, 1966). Social reinforcement was consequently interpreted by, among others, cognitive learning theorists as an information process (Bandura, 1977; Mahoney, 1974).

Praise, for example, reflects the attitude of the therapist or researcher, and the client or subject will try to behave in praiseworthy ways. Although these ideas are not shared by all learning theorists (e.g. Kanfer & Phillips, 1970), they surely question the assumption that therapeutic interaction is solely a conditioning process. Reinforcement contingencies are perceived by clients, who evaluate and actively respond to them.

Moreover, the concept of reinforcement is used somewhat falsely since it cannot be predicted whether the intended therapist behaviour indeed increases the probability of occurrence of the consequent client behaviour. It seems more appropriate to consider positive feedback. In a number of studies, positive feedback in conjunction with specific instructions appears to be the critical variable (Emmelkamp & Ultee, 1974; Leitenberg, Agras, Allen, Butz & Edwards, 1975). Although the concept of social reinforcement or positive feedback cannot be ignored, it is clear that it does not completely explain all therapist activity within the therapeutic process.

The importance of social reinforcement is based on the verbal influence of the therapist; however, Bandura (1971) emphasizes influence as the basis of modelling. In his social–cognitive theory, observing models plays an important role and, consequently, he sees a role for therapists in client change. In order for therapists to be able to adopt this role, it is necessary that they are viewed to a large extent as *attractive* and as having *high status* as experts. These are attributes that are also emphasized by the social psychological theories which will be detailed in Chapter 2. Identification with the therapist by the client is also necessary in terms of identifying with coping strategies.

Meichenbaum (1971) distinguished between *mastery* and *coping* models, in which the latter are perfect models for the client and the former are usually difficult to carry out and may even increase anxiety. According to Mahoney (1974), it follows that the therapist should try not to look perfect and devoid of problems but should show appropriate coping styles. It is in behavioural rehearsal and cognitive coping strategies that the influence from the principles of modelling is evident.

In sum, the client–therapist relationship can be looked at in two ways, either as a catalyst or as a therapeutic ingredient (Hoorens, 1986). The therapeutic relationship can have either a positive or a negative impact on the effectiveness of the diverse activities directed towards change. In this regard it is important to provide the client with explanations that enhance the credibility of the rationale for therapy. Therapeutic effectiveness is increased if activities are judged credible, relevant to the person's needs and acceptable in terms of response costs and if the therapist creates favourable outcome expectancies (Rosenthal, 1980).

The roles of the catalyst and therapeutic ingredients of the therapeutic relationship reciprocally influence each other. To the extent that therapists evoke a positive emotional response, they will be a stronger source of social reinforcement and, by the same token, will be more attractive as a role model, which in turn promotes client change.

Empirical findings

Despite the fact that, more recently, the therapeutic relationship has received increased attention in behaviour therapy, this has not resulted in systematic research. Although a number of descriptive studies of therapist behaviour have recently been published (e.g. Hahlweg, 1981), these should be seen rather as clinical reports and proposals from practice.

The first studies investigating the effects of specific behaviour patterns were carried out while investigating the effective ingredients of systematic desensitization. In these studies, the therapeutic style was experimentally manipulated and its effect on outcome was assessed. Morris and Suckerman (1974), for instance, reported that with a warm and friendly therapist, better results were obtained than with a "cold" therapist. The same research group failed to replicate the results, although it is questionable whether therapist behaviour can be reduced to such crude dimensions. These early studies have been criticized on the grounds of the method of treatment, their analogue character and the lack of relevance to clinical practice (DeVoge & Beck, 1978; McGlynn, 1976).

Moreover, differentiated studies and analyses have been reported. For instance, Alexander, Barton, Schiavo and Parsons (1976) investigated therapists' interpersonal skills in relation to outcome in the behavioural family treatment of delinquents. In this study, 21 therapists received a week's training in a semi-structured treatment program. After this training, the new therapists were rated by their trainers on a number of categories that may be summarized as: (1) relationship skills (skill to integrate affect and behaviour, warmth, humour) and (2) structuring skills (directiveness and assertiveness).

Following the training, each therapist treated one family. The results of this treatment were then related to the original therapist rating on the relationship skills. A multiple regression analysis showed that both categories of therapist behaviour explained 60% of the variance in outcome and that relationship skills were more important than structuring skills. The significance of this study lies in the fact that all therapists received a similar training, thus more or less guaranteeing similar competence in technical skills and in the differential application of the treatment. The authors conclude from their results that variables such as warmth and humour are only effective if the therapist is able to structure the sessions and have clear directives.

Ford (1978) examined the relationship between behaviour therapists' behaviour and the clients' perception of the therapeutic relationship. Thirty-two patients were randomly assigned to three therapeutic conditions for training in social competence. To assess the behaviour of the therapist, 9 minutes from a number of sessions were sampled and these segments were rated on 48 categories. Ford found that a nonverbal style, characterized by warmth, certainty, sincerity, control, relaxation and emotional responsiveness, corresponded with positive client ratings. This relationship between therapist behaviour and client perception was found in all three conditions and a positive perception by the client of the therapist was a good predictor of outcome.

Rabavilas, Boulougouris and Perissaki (1979) asked patients suffering from phobic and obsessive–compulsive disorders, who were treated using exposure in vivo, to judge their therapists on 16 variables pertaining to their style of treatment. Respect, understanding and interest were positively and significantly related to patient outcome, as were the style variables encouragement, challenge and explicitness. Satisfaction of dependency needs and permissiveness were negatively related.

Similar findings are reported by Schindler, Revenstorf, Hahlweg and Brengelman (1983) in behavioural marital therapy: couples who received contingency contracting and reciprocity training, and who showed long-term success, rated their therapists as more empathic, directive and active. Hoogduin and Duivenvoorden (1988) found that 80% of a group of 60 obsessive–compulsive patients could be accurately assigned to the failure or success group, based on a prediction model. In this model the variables depression, level of anxiety, motivation, intelligence, aggression, marital problems and delusional experiencing of their compulsion, were used as predictors of outcome. The clients who were incorrectly assigned to the failure group—and yet did improve—all reported experiencing a good therapeutic relationship.

In a previous study, Hoogduin (1986) studied 60 patients suffering from obsessive–compulsive disorders who were treated with exposure in vivo and response prevention. A significant correlation was found between outcome and the quality of the therapeutic relationship on the basis of scores on the

Dutch version of the *Relationship Inventory* (Barrett-Lennard, 1962; Lietaer, 1976) of both the clients and the therapists. Hoogduin, de Haan, Schaap and Severeijns (1988) replicated this association between the quality of the therapeutic relationship, measured at an earlier point in time, and outcome in a sample of 25 obsessive–compulsive patients. Emmelkamp and Van der Hout (1983), as well as Bennun and Schindler (1988), also reported a significant correlation between outcome and therapeutic relationship in the treatment of agoraphobic patients.

Comparison of different schools of psychotherapy

In the 1960s, Shostrom produced three famous films in which Carl Rogers, Fritz Perls and Albert Ellis interviewed the same client. These films were controversial because for the first time, prominent representatives of the different therapeutic schools publicly exposed their clinical work. Over the years, these films have become the object of research in a number of studies designed to identify and systematically specify aspects of therapeutic practice. Shostrom (1966) reported that Rogers scored highest on support and effective orientation, Perls was found to be the most intensive in experiencing contact, and Ellis the strongest on cognitive re-evaluation.

Meara, Shannon and Pepinsky (1979) reported clear differences between the three therapists using an analysis of different verbal styles. Based on the numbers of sentences as well as sentence length, Ellis showed the highest degree of complexity, followed by Perls and finally Rogers. The verbal behaviour of the client also showed significant differences between the three interviews.

Hill, Thames and Rardin (1979) analyzed the videotaped interviews using the Counsellor and Client Verbal Response Coding System (Hill, 1978). They were able to describe the different styles on a behavioural level: Rogers showed *minimal support, paraphrasing, interpretation* and *clarification*. Perls showed *directives* primarily, gave *information* and used *confrontation* and *interpretation* as well as *affirmation* for the client. Ellis appeared the most active, showing mostly *clarification, directives, interpretation* and *reformulation*.

In 1977, Shostrom produced another series of films. This time the therapists were Lazarus, Rogers and Shostrom himself, and again the therapists interviewed the same client. O'Dell and Bahmer (1981) analyzed the therapeutic relationship in this series and found that Lazarus spoke the most, expressed himself most clearly and included himself most often in the conversation; Rogers used the most positive words; while Shostrom was about halfway between these two therapists. When being interviewed by Rogers, the clients made the least negative formulations, but were more positive with Lazarus. Positive self-descriptions occurred to the same extent in the interviews with Lazarus and

Rogers, whereas negative self-descriptions occurred the least with Lazarus.

Lee and Uhleman (1984) analyzed transcripts of the same series of films with a category coding system developed by Friedlander (1982). Rogers' behaviour was the most clearly coded and was intended to encourage the client to speak. *Reflection, Support* and *Request for Information* categories constituted 89% of total activity. Shostrom and Lazarus were rather similar in their behaviour, although Lazarus showed more *Directive Guidance, Clarification, Request for Information* and *Interpretation*. Compared to the other two therapists, he showed less *Support* and *Reflection*, characterizing his style as active, directive and informative.

Mahrer, Nifakis, Abhukara and Sterner (1984) compared transcripts of therapy sessions by Wolpe, Rogers and Fagan with different clients. They were interested in the micro-strategies of each therapist, i.e. two consecutive utterances of each therapist. In this way, for each therapist, different behaviour sequences could be identified: Wolpe mainly used a series of information-seeking statements, sometimes followed or preceded by interpretations; Rogers mainly used reflections or simple assents, sometimes in combination with interpretations; Fagan, finally, showed a more varied pattern, consisting of information seeking, structuring and interpretation.

Schaap and Suntjes (1986) compared videotaped sessions of therapists from different schools used to train therapists. Ten sessions were transcribed and coded with the Verbal Response Mode (VRM; Stiles, 1979) coding system, to be described in Chapter 6. The results underscore the fact that the behaviour of therapists from different schools does indeed vary considerably, but also that many common elements can be identified. For instance, reflections, acknowledgements and interpretations were used by all therapists to a considerable degree. But perhaps the most interesting finding was that the behaviour within a therapeutic school varied according to the different types of sessions. For instance, the behaviour therapists showed reflections from a mere 3% in systematic desensitization (SD) to 13% during the session that the SD was planned. Similarly, 6% of all utterances were questions during the SD, whereas during a mediation therapy (a session with the parents focusing on behaviour change with their children) this was 14%.

These studies, and many others comparing prominent therapists, illustrate the characteristics of the different schools, but little can be extrapolated about the client's subjective experience since the repetition of the interviews with the same client must surely have an effect on behaviour. The differences found between the representatives of the different schools also cannot necessarily be generalized to other clients or to other representatives of the same therapeutic schools. These studies involve isolated interviews, comparable more or less to the first session in therapy, and in all cases can only be perceived as exploratory. The predictive power of studies that focus on a larger sample of clients and therapists is much greater and will be described in later chapters.

Sloane, Staples, Cristol, Yorkston and Whipple (1975) compared a total of 94 therapy cases conducted by three psychoanalysts and three behaviour therapists. Audiotaped segments of 4 minutes of the fifth session were rated by independent observers. The therapists of both schools showed the same emotional support and warmth. The behaviour therapists, however, had more intensive personal contact with their clients and were rated higher on empathy and congruence. They were generally more active, more vocal, gave more information and were more directive than the analysts.

Brunink and Schroeder (1979) compared audiotaped sessions of a total of 18 psychoanalysts, Gestalt and behaviour therapists. The Gestalt therapists were relatively easy to separate, whereas the psychoanalysts and behaviour therapists were similar in some of the categories. Gestalt therapists were more personal and more directive than the others but both behaviour therapists and the analysts tried more explicitly to facilitate communication and were more influenced by the clients. The behaviour therapists were rated as the most emotionally supportive and showed most flexibility and initiative. They were comparable with the analysts in interpretations but were more directive.

Comparable results were reported by Greenwald, Kornblith, Hersen, Bellack and Himmelhoch (1981). They studied two behaviour therapists and two analysts in their treatment of 20 depressive female patients. Three-minute samples from the fourth session and eighth session were analyzed, and the results indicated that the behaviour therapists were more directive and structuring and showed more initiative in establishing a more supportive climate. These results are similar to those reported by DeRubeis, Hollen, Evans and Bemis (1982), who also found this pattern of activities to be characteristic of behaviour therapists.

These latter studies, together with the analyses of the prominent representatives of the different schools, show that behaviour therapy has a characteristic style, which is different from other schools. Somewhat surprisingly, these studies indicate that behaviour therapists are rated higher on relationship variables such as empathy, unconditional positive regard and congruence than are Gestalt therapists and psychodynamic psychotherapists. These results clearly contradict the traditional stereotype of the "cold" and mechanistic behaviour therapist.

Conclusions

It is clear from the comparison of the theoretical principles of the different schools that each psychotherapeutic approach has systematized just one component. Client-centred therapy exclusively, and psychoanalysis to a lesser degree, has emphasized the relationship component, whereas behaviour therapy has historically emphasized technique. However, research on the different schools as clinically practiced presents a different picture, which provides provocative evidence for the importance of common factors. Many studies show that variation in the components of different approaches is more or less ignored in their theoretical formulation. Client-centred therapists do not refrain from such techniques as behavioural rehearsal or relaxation training, particularly in time-limited forms of treatment. Behaviour therapists show characteristics that theoretically would be associated with client-centred therapists' behaviour, suggesting that therapeutic change is only possible in the context of a therapeutic relationship. This does not mean that the ideal form of psychotherapy consists of the integration of the different elements from the different schools. The emphasis on common factors is often falsely associated with eclecticism: research on common factors in psychotherapy is directed towards the construction of a meta-theory of psychotherapy, whereas eclecticism implies the gathering of techniques from different psychotherapeutic approaches.

The concept of common factors represents a meta-model that describes the mechanism valid for all forms of psychotherapy. The further study of these factors will contribute to a better understanding of the therapeutic process and at the same time help to create a stronger connection between research and practice. Such a systematic study begins with an exact description of the therapeutic process. It is only then that it will be possible to explain specific effects as well as predict prognosis of an effect under specific conditions.

Since a description always implies a selection and must make use of verbal formulations, such progress is impossible without theoretical assumptions. This means that any empirical analysis should be preceded by a theoretical conceptualization (Reinecker, 1986; 1987). For this reason we will discuss social psychological formulations of therapeutic interaction in the next chapter.

2　Therapeutic change:
a process-oriented model

Introduction

Psychotherapy may be described as a complex cognitive, emotional, behavioural, and social process of change in an interpersonal context (Kanfer & Schefft, 1988). In the theoretical conceptualization and empirical test of factors that constitute this interpersonal context, behavioural psychotherapy is still in its infancy. Research within this school of psychotherapy has for decades focused on changing behaviour using particular techniques of intervention. And has done so at the cost of facing such fundamental questions as: Why do clients or patients make use of such techniques? Why would patients suddenly take steps they were unable to take on their own, although well aware of the necessity of doing so? Why do statements and instructions by the therapist move them? Why do clients attend to these observations and internalize them (Strong & Claiborn, 1982)?

The paradigms of conditioning are relevant for an essential part of treatment but learning theory is not sufficient to indicate how a comprehensive programme of change should be conducted (Kanfer & Grimm, 1980). In short, learning principles are not identical to the conditions under which learning takes place. The "particularity" of therapy is the establishment by the therapist of the conditions necessary for learning processes to get started and be fulfilled. The situation of clients is characterized by their inability to establish these conditions themselves. Therapy therefore also constitutes a goal-directed use of social influence as a condition for individual processes of learning.

What is lacking in behavioural psychotherapy is a process theory, firmly and empirically founded, that enables us to describe, clarify and predict changes that occur when taking into account this interpersonal aspect. Each systematic empirical analysis of events during psychotherapy does, however, presume a preliminary process model that enables the derivation of hypotheses and strategies of research. Using the results that are yielded, a theoretical model will be expanded, differentiated or modified. A single veridical process model can not be assumed. It is more a question of level of abstraction, that is, the level on which events are perceived as sufficiently precise to function as an element of a theoretical explanation or prognosis. A process model of behavioural psychotherapy can only be considered sufficiently precise if it enables the deduction of specific rules for the therapist on how to behave in particular situations. This means that one should strive for a conceptual framework that enables the operationalization of the strategies of social influence in such a way that they are testable on the level of concrete acts. Moreover, such a model should define the complementary roles of clients and therapists, and detail the phases of the therapy process. And, finally, it should specify the conditions under which learning can take place.

In research a social psychological direction has become increasingly more important during the last few years, in which psychotherapy is described as a process of social influence. It is the aim of this research to allow social psychological findings to be used in the explanation of the interpersonal events in psychotherapy. These theoretical principles may be useful for filling in the described gaps in the theoretical concept of behavioural psychotherapy.

In this chapter we attempt to bring together social psychological data, principles and theorems with the more empirical descriptions of change processes within behavioural psychotherapy. It should be pointed out that these social psychological formulations should not be perceived as substitutes for learning theoretical principles of change. Rather, they should serve to describe and explain the interpersonal context and the interaction between client and therapist, as well as the significance of these for individual change. Social psychological attempts at explaining psychotherapeutic change are to be perceived as a meta-theory, and are consequently to be related to the therapeutic process specific for behavioural psychotherapy. Kanfer and Grimm (1980) described a phase model for what goes on in behavioural psychotherapy. In this model the interpersonal aspects are explicitly included. In connection with this behavioural model, these social psychological theorems can be considered to be the conceptual framework for an empirical analysis of the interpersonal aspects in psychotherapy.

Actually, attempts at integrating social psychological research and the practice of behavioural psychotherapy are not new. Wolpe and Lazarus (1966) emphasized the significance of the client–therapist interaction for successful change. Later, the voices in favour of an integration of social psychological explanation models in the theory development within behavioural psychotherapy became increasingly strong (e.g. Kanfer & Phillips, 1970; Wilson & Evans, 1977). A real integration has thus far not been achieved, since a unified theory for behavioural psychotherapy is lacking (e.g. Kazdin, 1979). Consequently, the attempts at integration remain thus far on the level of single attempts (e.g.

DeVoge & Beck, 1978; Feldmann, 1976). A fundamental problem in the translation of social psychological models into the clinical sphere is the fact that a single social psychological theory is also lacking. Social psychology is composed of a heterogeneous multitude of mini-theories, concepts and problems that are in dire need of further formulation and study (e.g. Brehm, 1976). As a result, the more recent attempts at translating consist of combinations of various social psychological theories, in order to do justice to the complex chain of events in therapeutic change (e.g. Johnson & Matross, 1977; Strong, 1978; Strong & Claiborn, 1982). The difficulty, in search of theorems that in terms of theory of science are parsimonious and enable an empirical testing of their clinical derivations, is made abundantly clear by Strong (1982), who reviewed a decade of research in this area. This review resulted in a formulation of a network of heterogeneous assumptions from such diverse constructs as social exchange, social power, cognitive dissonance, attribution and reactance. As a result, many propositions in these integrative attempts remain speculative and need the support and correction of empirical results. The immediate translation of empirical findings from social psychological research into the clinical sphere is also problematic because of the analogue character of many social psychological studies. The problems regarding the theories, their integration and their translation do not permit an elaborated theory at this point in time (e.g. Heppner & Claiborn, 1989; Kanfer, 1984). What is presented, however, is a theoretical framework from which strategies for the systematic study of interpersonal events may be derived.

Contributions from social psychology: therapy as a process of social influence

Brehm and Smith (1986) showed the historical connection between the area of social and clinical psychology. Social psychologists have attempted to explain the social aspect of psychotherapy with their theorems. Originally, these attempts only contained assumptions that can be described as personality-related and static (Johnson & Matross, 1977). A literature search yields a mass of research on the qualities of therapists that define their attractiveness, credibility and expert status. Only during the 1970s did this change. Social influence was no longer understood simply as the function of static and discrete qualities of the influencer (persuader) and the influenced (persuaded), but as the product of a changing relationship between two individuals (Johnson & Matross, 1977; Strong & Matross, 1973). With the pioneering work of Strong (1968), therapeutic change was conceived in a social psychological perspective as the result of a process of interpersonal influence. Perhaps the most extensive presentation of this perspective is provided by Strong and Claiborn (1982), which still determines the conceptualization used presently (see Heppner & Claiborn, 1989).

In the following pages the social psychological conceptualization of the process of therapy and therapeutic relationship will be described on the basis of the work of Janis (1982), Strong and Claiborn (1982), Dorn (1986) and Maddux, Stoltenberg and Rosenwein (1987). For a more extensive review of the fundamental social psychological theorems we refer to this literature. We will, nevertheless, describe in short the most important social psychological principles of relevance to psychotherapy for the reader not acquainted with social psychology.

The social psychological conceptualization of psychotherapy as a process of social influence can be perceived as a further development of the search for common factors (Van Kalmthout et al, 1985). Within this meta-theory an attempt is made to specify how the roles of client and therapist are to be characterized, the form in which the therapeutic relationship is established, the way in which this relationship can prepare for or effectuate therapeutic change and, finally, the disturbances in the process of change that can occur (resistance).

Relevant theories from social psychology

Exchange theory

Exchange theory (Thibaut & Kelley, 1959) within a behavioural process model is a particularly suitable theoretical framework, since it constitutes an attempt to apply the explanatory categories of behavioural theory to the analysis of social behaviour. In so doing, it is able to arrive at the closest possible connection between behaviour and interaction theory.

Social interaction is considered as an exchange of tangible or intangible goods (which may be rewarding or expensive) with feelings, attitudes and acts (Homans, 1961). With regard to quantity or value, these goods are in principle operationalized, such that it is possible to calculate profit, cost or utility within any interaction. Homans considers the following goods as utilities: love, status and information. Costs of goods such as time, energy or material investment are construed according to the following principles: the behaviour of one person is followed by either a reward or a punishment; the more often, and the more subjectively valued an activity is rewarded, the more likely a person is to show this same activity in the future. However, continuous use of the same reward makes it less valuable, resulting in satiation. If a certain expected reward does not occur, or if a particular activity is punished, then the person will respond aggressively or with irritation, and the outcome will be experienced as reinforcing. This idea is, for instance, expanded in a context of family interaction and relationships by Patterson (1976) who used the illustrative title 'The aggressive child: *Victim* and *architect* of a coercive system'.

Exchange theorists suppose that each person is striving towards maximization of reward (Thibaut & Kelley, 1959). It is only possible for two persons to begin a permanent social relationship, if the investment is low relative to the outcome of the relationship. If the ratio between investment and outcome will change in an unfavourable direction, then the social relationship will be dissolved. In principle it should be possible to calculate at each moment the outcome of the relationship. Thibaut and Kelley (1959), moreover, assumed that each partner will measure outcome of the interaction using an internal criterion. The level of this criterion constitutes the minimal standard at which the person evaluates the relationship. This means the amount and type of rewards and investments a person can expect, measured by that which he or she thinks is reasonable, based on his or her experience. Moreover, people also measure the outcome of any interaction with a level of comparison with alternatives. If the outcome of the internal level of comparison lies clearly below the alternative level, then the relationship will be dissolved.

Inside the relationship each behaviour is a link in a continuous chain of interaction. Each behavioural unit of one person is caused by the behaviour of the other person but it also has an impact on the following behaviour of that person. Both partners influence each other's behaviour (circular causality). The content of social exchange is described as resources. Foa and Foa (1980) presented a classification into six types of resources that may be described in a two-dimensional system.

The first dimension refers to the concreteness versus symbolization of the resource, i.e. the extent to which the reinforcer is material or symbolic. The second dimension refers to the particularism versus universality of the resource. This refers to the extent that a resource is connected with a particular person or depends on the person as a provider. Foa and Foa (1980) emphasized not only the classification value of these categories but also the functional character of the system. They considered it more probable that resources are exchanged that are close together in their classification than resources that are further apart or opposite. In criticism of this principle, the same act or behaviour can be associated with different resources by different persons. Moreover, the configuration only refers to positive resources. One could argue that it would be sensible to construct such a taxonomy for punishments and investments as well.

By means of these resources, two persons in a relationship control each other. The extent of this control is a function of the dependence of the persons on these resources, i.e. how high they evaluate them. In other words, the extent of the dependence of person A on person B is a function of the strength of A's needs and of the consequent available resources of person B. Need is in this formulation conceived as a perceived shortage of psychological or physical qualities such as attraction, information, experience, food, security, status. The resource of person B is the capacity to prepare such qualities. The extent of the dependence is a function of the strength of the need and the extent of the resource that is connected with this need. A decisive role is played by perception. It is not important if B is aware of his or her own resources. Dependence originates from the estimation by A.

Exchange theories have had a pervasive influence on social psychological theory construction because they make social interaction analysable from the perspective of negotiation and exchange. Interaction, seen as exchange, in principle opens the possibility of empirically studying social behaviour. It also pulls social behaviour towards learning theory and behaviourism. It is exactly this point that has led to a great deal of criticism. The connection with behaviourism is illegitimate, that is to say, since the introduced concepts are less exact than originally used in the operant tradition. Moreover, essential ideas of Skinner, e.g. about reinforcement schedules, are ignored. However, the strongest critique is formulated against the picture that emerges from this theory. By introducing the first postulate of economics as the maxim for relationships, calculation and profit are introduced. Even if it is obviously impossible to parry such critique completely, one should emphasize that exchange theory uses these concepts as analogies (Chadwick-Jones, 1976). Another point of critique concerns the problem of operationalizing such constructs as investment, profit, and reward. Usually, only a *post hoc* analysis is possible.

All in all, however, if one also considers other necessary functions of social theories in one's judgement, for instance its heuristic value, then social exchange theories have achieved much in terms of integration and organization of knowledge, as well as in the mediation of insights and interpretation.

Social power and influence

Because of the described interdependence that interacting persons have on the present resources of each other, the condition for yielding social influence is created. Based on the needs regarding the resources of the other, the dependent person is prepared to establish, to change or to keep up the relationship. If necessary, he or she will even change his or her own behaviour or attitudes in order to defend the relationship. Social power is therefore described as the capability attributed to a person to influence cognitive or behavioural aspects of another on the basis of their power over and accessibility to particular resources. The power range is consequently comprised of acts, decisions and ideas of the other person in the interaction. The extent of the dependence is defined by the sensitivity of one person regarding the proposal for the definition of the relationship by the other person. The ability of person A to influence person B requires B's dependency on A with respect to certain resources that B needs in order to attain his goals (Cartwright, 1959).

In their differentiation of means of power, French and Raven (1959) distinguished between power by reinforcement (reward) and coercive power. These are based on legitimation, identification, knowledge and information. The constructs of dependency and social power are operationally linked to the observed behavioural change of a person that results from the request by another person. Social influence is accordingly observable, successful execution of power.

Strong and Matross (1973) sketched a model of the psychotherapeutic process, based on social psychological research on attitude change and influence. The processes by which the therapist influences his client, they label as social power. The essence of this social power is formed by the experience of the client as dependent on the therapist. This experience is generated by the relationship that the client forms between his personal and interpersonal needs, and the abilities of the therapist to satisfy these needs. The way in which the client experiences this relationship can be over- and underestimated and is, moreover, dependent on the way the client experiences this relationship in his or her contacts with other people. In this model, the expectation of the client to be able to satisfy certain needs via the therapist and the therapy has a central position. According to Strong and Matross, it is essentially the power relationship between client and therapist that enables this influence through therapy.

The construct of social power can be divided into five themes, labelled power bases. Each power base refers to a relationship between a particular need of the client and a particular quality of the therapist. These five power bases, labelled expert, referent, legitimate, informational and ecological, will be discussed as follows.

Expert power base   A person feels at a standstill with his or her problems. The present situation cannot continue. Attempts to solve the problem have been unsuccessful, which may have even resulted in more problems in terms of anxiety, stress and lack of well-being. Then, the person enters psychotherapy because of experiencing the need to achieve his or her goals against reduced costs, and because he or she believes the therapist has special knowledge and the expertise to help him or her. Next to the need for help, the expert power base is determined by the extent to which the client perceives the therapist as a person who can help by his or her specialized knowledge about psychological processes, interpersonal relationships and therapeutic skills.

Referent power base   This power base is originally based on the theory of cognitive dissonance (Festinger, 1954). The problems that lead a client to decide to begin therapy are often the result of an experience of inconsistency between his or her behaviour and values or norms. This inconsistency is a subjective experience and, more often than not, is based on social comparisons and not so much on objective perceptions. This implies that the client in interaction with others will try to reduce this psychological inconsistency. The therapist wins referent power to the extent that he or she is considered attractive, is empathetic with the experiences of the client, and offers him or herself as comparison material and a standard measure. The client will tend to let him or herself be influenced to overcome the experience of inconsistency. This description is very similar to the ideas formulated by Frank (1973) and has been labelled the demoralization of the client. In this way, referent power base refers to a personal relationship from whom the client distills those elements that will help him to experience himself as increasingly integrated (Corrigan, Dell, Lewis & Schmidt, 1980).

By formulating 12 key variables in three phases of the treatment process that determine the degree of referent power of counsellors and therapists as agents of change, Janis (1982) described the actual elements from the standpoint of the therapist. The three phases are: building up, using, and retaining referent power. The following variables are distinguished by Janis (1982):

Building up referent power

1 By encouraging clients to make self-disclosure.
2 By giving positive feedback.
3 By using self-disclosures to give insight and cognitive restructuring.

Using referent power

4 By making directive statements or endorsing specific recommendations regarding actions the client should carry out.
5 By eliciting commitment to the recommended course of action.
6 By attributing the norms being endorsed to a respected secondary group.
7 By giving selective positive feedback.
8 By giving communications and training procedures that build up a sense of personal responsibility.

Retaining referent power

9 By giving reassurances that the therapist will continue to maintain an attitude of positive regard.
10 By making arrangements for phone calls, exchange of letters or other forms of communication that foster hope for future contact, real or symbolic, at the time of terminating face-to-face meetings.
11 By giving reminders that continue to foster a sense of personal responsibility.
12 By building up the client's self-confidence about succeeding without the aid of the therapist.

We will return to these and similar variables in a later section on the process model as well as in later chapters in which strategies are formulated and illustrated to motivate the client to change.

Legitimate power base   This third base is founded in the acceptance of the client of the therapeutic relationship and its role division. This base is increasingly more important to the extent that the client's involvement in the therapeutic process increases. The decision to accept treatment and to participate actively in the therapeutic process will lessen the client's resistance against suggestions from the therapist. Resistance would be dissonant with the client's participation, according to self-perception and cognitive dissonance theories (Strong & Matross, 1973; Tennen, Rohrbach, Press & White, 1981).

Informational power base   This power base will become more important to the extent that the client needs information about how his or her goals may be reached, and to the extent that the therapist is perceived as a person who has access to this information. The authors distinguish this base from the expert power base in that the therapist can give the client information or material that will influence his behaviour outside the sessions.

Ecological power base   This power base refers to the influence of the therapist by mediation of the client's environment. It constitutes an indirect way of influencing the client to change certain aspects of his or her life. The client may be encouraged to go to school, to engage in social contacts, to get a divorce. Important aspects of this power base are constituted by getting the family involved, by providing information to spouse and family, and by instructing the family to respond in certain ways. Research confirms the positive effect of social support on engaging in treatment, on continuing treatment and on successfully ending treatment (Miller, 1985).

Next to social power the authors distinguish between two powers in the client that may oppose this influencing process by the therapist: resistance and opposition. *Resistance* refers to noncompliant behaviour of the client that has its origin in the nature of the interaction with the therapist. The way the therapist engages in influencing attempts is considered by the client to be inappropriate. This may be the case when a therapist does not respond with the corresponding power base. For instance, a therapist with a high expert base and low reference base will increase the probability of noncompliant or resistive behaviour if he or she chooses an intimate and personal way of influencing ("I think it is necessary to...") in contrast to if he or she chooses a more impersonal way ("In the frame of treatment is is necessary that...").

Opposition refers to noncompliant behaviour or resistive behaviour of the client that finds its origin in the content of the influence attempt. The opposition is directed to the nature of the change. A change from situation A to situation B can be anxiety-provoking, when the client has reached an equilibrium. Opposition will be particularly strong if situation A satisfies needs of the client that are not satisfied by B any more, or if the basis for the need has disappeared. For instance, by being unassertive, a client may be able to avoid fights with spouse, family or colleagues. To motivate the client to exhibit assertive behaviour, the therapist has to address illogical cognitions and values, which will have to be changed.

In a dyadic relationship there never exists complete unilateral dependency. If no desired resource can be detected, no enduring interaction with that person will result. The greater the dependency, the more robust the relationship is and the more likely it is that incongruence will effectuate a behavioural change in one or both interaction partners. Incongruence is defined as the discrepancy between the actual relationship and the personal definition of the relationship. The relationship between dependency and influence can vary greatly. Since the more powerful person is also to a certain degree dependent on the other person, a total influencibility of the dependent person can never be reached. Therefore, the usual script for building a relationship is a continual negotiation on both sides, with the end result that it gives more to the more powerful person than to the other. Change can be a move in the dependent person's strategy to gain more control in the relationship, since change represents a resource for the more powerful person. Change will, therefore, occur in the direction of the need of the more powerful person and may be considered an attempt of the dependent person to minimize the power advantage.

Change is, however, not guaranteed by a power lead alone. It also depends on the type of change that is proposed. The dependent person might experience a discrepancy between the change proposed by the more powerful person and his own definition of the relationship. Change in the desired direction might be too costly and painful. If the cost exceeds the social power of the other person, the dependent person may refuse the change, even if the relationship gets into danger. Also, the comparison level is important here. If the person is convinced that he will be able to get the same resources for less costs, he will be prepared to risk the actual relationship.

Theory of cognitive dissonance

The theory of cognitive dissonance is one of a number of dissonance theories and goes back to the fundamental concepts of balance theory, proposed by Heider (1944). According to this theory, persons are directed to organize their convictions and attitudes consistently with their behaviour, and to keep this balance. Two elements (X and Y) are considered consonant if one element follows from the other. X and Y are dissonant if from the existence of one element the opposite of the other follows. If a person perceives that his own behaviour contradicts his own attitudes and convictions, then there exists a condition of cognitive inconsistency. This condition is experienced as unpleasant, and will generate tension. The person is then motivated to change his attitudes and convictions into a consistent and, therefore, tensionless relationship. This will, however, only be the case under the condition that the inconsistent cognitions are relevant to behaviour. The strength of the dissonance is a result of the ratio between the number of dissonant and the number of consonant relationships. It is, moreover, determined by the personal meaning or valuation of the elements. In turn, the strength of the dissonance will determine the height of the motivation. In later versions of cognitive dissonance theory, the significance of the voluntary engagements and of nonambivalent commitment is introduced. Only when a person has committed himself by his behaviour will he experience dissonance and will he try to reduce it. Three strategies for reducing dissonance are distinguished: (a) cognitive change about own behaviour change, (b) cognitive change about the influence of the environment, and (c) the addition of new cognitive elements. The type of strategy that is chosen depends on the cognitive structure of the individual.

For an induction of dissonance to be successful, the person has to proclaim clearly the desire for change and commit him- or herself voluntarily by the formulation of goals (Kiesler, 1971). Commitment is defined as a psychological condition that occurs when a person knows that he or she will show a particular behaviour, is presently showing that behaviour or will show that behaviour in the future. The corresponding behaviour is usually public, since such behaviour guarantees that the person knows that he or she has agreed on that behaviour. The probability that a commitment will result in attitude change depends on the fact that the person feels responsible. Personal responsibility is best created by presenting alternatives. The conditions for such commitments are favourable in cases in which the client comes of his or her own free will. He or she already has shown a step in seeking help. Inconsistency would be greater if he or she would decline further co-operation (effort justification) (Cooper & Axsom, 1982).

On the one hand, the dissonance theory has had much resonance and has stimulated a great number of studies. On the other hand, in such studies the expected results were often not reached. This had to do with the fundamental measurement problems, since it is assumed or implied that the cognitive structure of an individual is transparent, in order to be able to define the strength of the dissonance. The problem is to delineate an individual cognitive element, to measure the importance of this element, and to define the number of consonant and dissonant elements. Nevertheless, dissonance theory is plausible and useful, since phenomena are described that reflect ideas from everyday psychology. On the other hand, phenomena are described that can be derived from older psychological theories, and that can be considered to be experimentally founded.

Attribution and reactance

Everybody has a need to understand the external and internal world, and in particular their social environment and emotions. One tries to achieve the construction of consistent images of reality, in order to derive from this construction feelings of security and control. This also enables the person to better respond towards changes in his or her environment. Attribution theory assumes that people continually construct a consistent and understandable world by means of attributing meaning and causes to events (Kelley & Thibaut, 1978). Attributions are made on the basis of successes or failures of earlier attributions.

Attributions can take on many forms and can be characterized in many ways. However, a number of dimensions can be formulated. An important dimension is between internal and external attributions. In the former, the cause is sought within the person, whereas in the latter form, external circumstances or other persons are seen as the cause of important events. Such attributions obviously influence the ways persons attach meaning to their problems and the strategies that are chosen to solve these problems.

Attributions can serve different functions. These functions are sometimes interpreted as explanations of or as motives for which people make attributions (Hewstone, 1983). The following functions are mentioned in the literature:

1 *Control, security and predictability.* For instance, stereotyping is a method of making one's world (and the people in it) more predictable and controllable. Also self-reproach can function as a kind of protection, a buffer against a threatening world where things can happen at random.
2 *Protection of a feeling of self-esteem.* External attributes for failures and internal attributions for successes may be explained from this need.
3 *Impression management or the creation of a favourable image.* In interaction with others, attributions are presented with the aim of presenting a favourable image of oneself.

These functions do refer to fundamental needs. This implies that if people are confronted with opposite attributions, they will tend to resist. What is implied by the term resistance could to a large extent be derived from this.

Attributions, once established, may be changed under a number of conditions. This process is called re-attribution and may occur in cases of:

- unknown, uncertain or unclear situations,
- the new attribution gives a sense of greater control,
- lack of social support for the old attribution,
- strong support for the new attribution,
- strong authority attributed to the definer,
- a warm relationship with the definer,
- remaining powerless in a particular situation,
- plausibility of the new attribution,
- the old attribution not fitting into the stereotype way of attributing.

Fundamental propositions about the process of social influence

The client's situation

Frank (1985) described demoralisation as the fundamental characteristic of clients regardless of presenting symptoms. Demoralisation is the outcome of failing skills and capacities, loss of self-confidence, feelings of estrangement and hopelessness. This condition is captured perhaps more accurately by Bandura's (1977) *self-efficacy model* where expectations play an important role. Bandura (1977) distinguished between outcome expectations and efficacy expectations.

Outcome expectations are defined as the person's estimation that a particular behaviour will lead to a desired outcome. The *efficacy expectation*, in contrast, refers to the person's conviction that he/she is able to produce that behaviour that is necessary to attain the desired outcome. The distinction between both types of expectations is therefore important, since individuals may be absolutely sure that a certain behaviour will lead to a desired condition but, if they doubt their ability to carry out the necessary behaviour effectively, this knowledge will have no influence on the eventual outcome. In other words, although the person might know which behaviours are necessary to solve a problem, he/she might feel unable to apply this solution and will therefore refrain from even attempting to do so. Recognizing personal helplessness will lead persons to seek alternative problem solutions.

The client's situation, as characterized by being incapable of reaching the desired goals, leads to the search for professional help. This will presumably consist of information and guidance, that are not available to clients in their natural social environment. Finding a person to whom power of commanding and providing consequent resources can be ascribed will be the goal of this search.

The therapist's situation

The therapist is socially recognized as an expert in solving emotional problems and as such, this social sanction is expressed in special training and is emphasized by, for example, academic titles. These attributes generate the expectation that the therapist commands the knowledge and opportunities to help other people solve their problems, thus reinforcing their personal social status resources as helpers. The status of an expert is important in mediating credibility and trustworthiness (Johnson & Matross, 1977). Reviewing a large number of studies, Corrigan et al. (1980) concluded that therapists, by way of their social role alone, are ascribed a high status as experts and that this role expectation is even greater than the impact of their perceived expertise or attractiveness. However, this only applies at the beginning of treatment and, if the therapist appears incompetent in the further course of treatment, then the original legitimate power is undermined (see also Heppner & Claiborn, 1989).

About the needs of therapists—and therefore the resources that clients have at their disposal—one can only speculate. Henry, Sims and Spray (1971) studied the motives for people to enroll in the helping professions. Psychologists were characterized mostly by an interest in understanding psychological phenomena. This is supported by Blaser (1981). Therapists, interviewed about their main reason to take a patient on in therapy, mentioned that their primary interest was the patient. Rated second was the desire to help the patient. A charitable attitude is therefore more or less pronounced (Marston, 1984). Apart from motives such as these, however, there exists the professional honour of attaining success with clients. Improvement as such, as well as the connected expression of thankfulness, could well constitute the resources provided by clients. Furthermore, helping has become the therapist's existential foundation and means of existence, in which material reward plays an important role.

Establishing the relationship

Clients who freely seek therapy will choose a therapist on the basis of recommendations, possibly the theoretical approach or their institutional affiliation. The decision to enter therapy will only be taken if there are no other people in their social network to whom similar resources can be ascribed and who could be used with less investment and cost. The decision to seek professional help and the actual step of referral imply an important investment and are the first signs of commitment. The decision whether to accept a client will depend on the therapist's competence, the client's psychological state, and the therapist's perception of treatment success (Feldman, 1976). It may also be determined by therapists' desire to take only clients in therapy with whom success can be predicted. Once engaged in treatment, both will try to establish a congruent and stable relationship (Strong & Claiborn, 1982); however, incongruence will occur if one or both partners experience a discrepancy within the relationship. Stability refers to the probability of maintaining or breaking the relationship and also depends on interpersonal congruence. Unstable and incongruent relationships can be used positively if the opportunity for behaviour change does not threaten the therapeutic relationship. Social power in treatment relationships can be defined through the therapist's access to and knowledge of expert information. Usually this information is required and valued by clients, yet often they do not wish to expend great costs in following this advice. The social power is further strengthened if the client cannot gain valued information and help from anyone else.

Relationship and change

Attitudes and behaviour are the objects of change. In addition to a behavioural repertoire, clients have a particular set of attitudes, i.e. an accepted view of the world. Positive outcome depends on facilitating changes in the client's personal assumptions. These assumptions relate to their understanding of the origin of their disturbance, knowledge about alternatives, and the modifiability of social norms. Clients are dependent on the therapist's resources and therefore value maintaining the relationship. In order not to endanger this relationship, they are usually prepared to accept information or to change their attitudes and behaviour to a certain extent. The prospect of a favourable outcome is enhanced if a client seeks help voluntarily, as opposed to say a court order. Declining help in this stage of therapy would appear to be inconsistent with the already recognised need and willingness to change ("effort justification": Cooper & Axsom, 1982). An illustration of the effect of "being in therapy" is often encountered in reports (sometimes substantive) about improvements in placebo and control groups (Sloane et al., 1975), particularly if a credible rationale is provided. Clients can reduce their incongruence within the therapeutic relationship by improving. However, this in turn will result in an inconsistency in cognitive structure, indicating the necessity of further change.

It has already been pointed out that power and influence are initial resources that clients attribute to therapists. If titles and other status symbols determine the choice of the therapist, then the therapist will have to behave in a way that is consistent with these attributes. The probability of influence is therefore a product of the mutual relationship and depends on the form of the relationship. Therapists can influence clients as long as they have methods or resources that enable clients to reach personal goals; the more these goals are valued by the client, the greater is the influence of the therapist. Strong and Claiborn (1982) represented this process in a phase model.

During the *first* phase of treatment, the therapist enters the client's frame of reference in order to understand it more precisely. By showing this acceptance and understanding, the client begins to trust the therapist and will accept the role division.

During the *second* phase, therapists move back to their own frame of reference and introduce new information and explanations or propose changes that will imply a tolerable level of discrepancy. This will involve offering the client an explanatory model that will generate ideas about how to reduce the discrepancy. This model implies assumptions about the origins and control of behaviour patterns and enables criteria of change to be identified. Clients will be able to accept this model if it is not too far removed from their present level of understanding (Claiborn, Ward & Strong, 1981; Strong, Wambach, Lopez & Cooper, 1979) and, in so doing, reinforce the therapist as expert. It will also provide a framework of goals and course of treatment.

During treatment, the therapist needs to introduce proposals for change, yet these will inevitably be discrepant with the client's present way of functioning. Obviously, the level of discrepancy that is introduced needs to be tolerable, so that the therapeutic relationship is not threatened. Freedman and Fraser (1966) were able to show that clients who successfully complied with small assignments were later more likely to embark on assignments requiring more investment. The successful therapist perceives the changes that are feasible and continues until the full extent of possible change has been reached.

It is important that clients commit themselves to goals even if these lead to dissonance. In addition, clients can choose this commitment voluntarily and be informed about the negative consequences of this choice. In this situation, individual responsibility increases, which in turn is the necessary condition for dissonance and the consequent attempts to reduce it (Brehm, 1976; Feldman, 1976). If this is successful, then the client will gradually change attitudes and behaviour so as to achieve therapeutic goals. Once the client is able to achieve outcome independently, the reliance on the therapist's resources will decrease.

Consequently, therapists will choose at each moment in time that form of an utterance that is directed towards these goals. In each interaction sequence therapists will focus on particular subgoals and will make an estimate of the actual status in the discourse. The comparison of subgoal and actual state of affairs will generate a particular intention for the next step and the behavioural manner of achieving that goal. The therapist's behaviour will have an impact on the client's experiences and a consequent behavioural response.

The therapeutic discourse is therefore a therapist-planned, systematic process of verbalized attitude changes of the client.

The verbalization of changing cognitive frames has different functions. First, there exists no other way for the therapist to be able to perceive changes in the client during the session. Second, the articulation signifies a cognitive process in which each message presents a new perspective or intention, implying a commitment in the above sense.

The more anxiety and inhibitions are present in the client, the less simple will be the explanations by the therapist that will lead to an attitude change. This highlights the importance of a strategic approach on the part of the therapist. Strong (1982) considered the most important feature of the therapeutic situation to be for therapists to behave in an unexpected way in their utterances and positions (cf. the "asocial response"; Beier, 1966). This means that dissonance is not only generated by the content of a message, but by its form as well. Often the humorous, provocative or paradoxical form of a message will enable clients to attend to, listen to and process the content. So, only if a sufficient level of attentiveness of the client is reached, will messages cognitively be processed, established and result in behavioural changes. Particularly these aspects of cognitive processing have been increasingly studied and specified during the last years (Cacioppo, Petty & Stoltenberg, 1985; McNeill & Stoltenberg, 1989). We should add, however, that social psychological research does not yet answer the important question as to how achieve this cognitive processing with different clients and the consequences for the actual therapy process (e.g. Heppner & Claiborn, 1989).

The social influence of the therapist will change in the course of treatment to the extent that the relationship changes. During the *third* phase, the relationship changes to one of congruence when the original needs of the client are satisfied and no new discrepancy is introduced. Clients will simply have less need of therapists. Consequently, therapists will have less social influence and the relationship will become more congruent. The congruent but unstable relationship will as a result end.

The origin of resistance

The above section outlines the ideal course of treatment, yet in clinical practice therapists often encounter disturbances, that are labelled as *resistance*. Although this term has its roots in psychoanalytic therapy, with a special meaning, it describes a behavioural pattern that occurs in all forms of treatment. It may be defined as the extent to which the client opposes change attempts by the therapist (Davison, 1973). According to Strong and Matross (1973), if no force would be present in clients that opposes change, clients would be able to develop independently and there would be no need to seek therapeutic help.

On the basis of the fundamental principles of client–therapist interaction described above, a number of different causes for the generation of counter-forces and disturbances in the ideal course of treatment may be derived. Four determining sources may be distinguished: the person of the client, the person of the therapist, their common interaction, and the environment of the client (Baekeland & Lundwall, 1975).

Client variables

The client's recognition of need and the voluntary decision to enter therapy are essential ingredients of the model. This is a precondition to receiving perceived therapist resources and, by the same token, a condition for responding to social influences. If clients enter therapy involuntarily, then change will occur only if the therapist succeeds in creating the need, e.g. by increasing suffering, by diminishing secondary gains or by involving a third party such as the spouse (see the following chapters for illustrations). However, there are other grounds that may make it difficult for a person to adopt the role of a dependent client. If clients exhibit an interaction style that does not permit a dependent relationship, they will consequently try and control the therapist by other means than behaviour change.

Therapist variables

If therapists show behaviour that is incongruent with their status as experts then they will undermine the conditions that facilitate social influence; an example is too much therapist self-disclosure. DeVoge and Beck (1978) and Keijsers, Schaap, Keijsers and Hoogduin (1990) have described these phenomena on the basis of the interpersonal diagnosis of Leary (1957) and Carson (1969). Furthermore, changes proposed by the therapist are likely to result in client dissonance, yet it is possible that the therapist will fail in this goal by underestimating the client's level of tolerance and may demand too much or too little.

Relationship variables

If the explanatory models or therapeutic goals of client and therapist do not match, the expectations of the client and the resources of the therapist will not be fulfilled. If the therapist proposes client change that demands too high a cost, these changes will be opposed because they induce uncomfortable levels of anxiety or shame. This may refer to themes or exercises within the session, as well as homework assignments in between sessions. There may also be resistance if the changes are perceived as coercion, which will undermine commitment and compliance (Brehm, 1976).

Environmental variables

Significant others in the client's environment can also obstruct deployment of the therapist's resources and the change process by questioning the expert status of the therapist, the rationale of treatment and, consequently, the relationship. Moreover, others may respond with aversive behaviour to changes in the clients' behaviour, thereby preventing the generation of new attitudes and behaviour: the cost of change is thus increased. Clients could also, as a consequence, seek alternative therapeutic relationships if they believe they are able to find the same resources at reduced cost. This will be the case particularly if the "illness theory" of therapist and clients differ.

The literature often implies that the occurrence of resistance is the exception and that it should be dealt with or avoided since it is likely to lead to dropout or treatment failure. However, the opposite seems to be true. O'Dell (1982), for instance, found that only 25% of the clients of parent trainers were considered "easy" to work with. So, resistance might be more the rule than the exception. We consider the following pragmatic definition of resistance a good starting point for the generation of strategies to handle resistance:

> Resistance is a sign that the therapist is not handling that particular client in the right way (and by the same token as a sign that the therapist should search for alternative means of handling the client).

We will return to this issue more extensively in Part II of this volume.

The phase model of Kanfer and colleagues

The social psychological principles allow for the description of psychotherapy as a process of social influence. The therapist directs the interaction with the client in such a way that the client accepts the intervention techniques and applies them between sessions. Social influence together with the systematic and time-limited application of therapeutic techniques enables the client to progress stepwise in the direction of the therapeutic goals.

Kanfer and Grimm (1980) formulated a process model that constitutes the bridge between assumptions of social influence and the structuring of the therapy process that is typical for behavioural psychotherapy. Therapy is considered a cooperative process of problem solving. The structure and the conduction of a behaviourally oriented therapy is mainly described in the literature as, however, the decision process of therapists during assessment and during the planning of treatment (i.e. Brinkman, 1978; Schulte, 1974). Kanfer and Grimm (1980), explicitly added interpersonal aspects, by describing seven phases in the ideal course of treatment. Although the different phases are often difficult to distinguish in reality, they represent an attempt at conceptualizing the progress of the therapeutic influence from the inception of the therapeutic relationship, over the application of techniques of intervention, towards the dissolution of the therapeutic bond. The model has been extended by Kanfer and Schefft (1988) and Kanfer, Reinecker and Schmelzer (1990), who specified for each phase the therapeutic goals and the ways of reaching these goals. The consequent strategic deliberations and advice for the therapist have been developed. What is still lacking though is an empirically defined indication of the particular therapist behaviour that should be shown in each problematic situation.

For an extensive description of this model we refer to Kanfer and Schefft (1988). We will limit ourselves to the description of concrete behavioural features that may be derived from empirical research thus far conducted within the different schools of psychotherapy. This research will be extensively described in the following chapters. In this chapter we will try and operationalize the therapist behaviours necessary in fulfilling the conditions of each of the seven phases. In other words, with the use of which behavioural forms can the therapist attain the necessary effect in the client?

Phase 1: role definition and the development of a therapeutic alliance

The primary task in this phase is the establishment of a trustful relationship as a precondition for any method of social influence. According to Strong and Claiborn (1982), therapists try to move within the conceptual frame of clients and accept their presentation of reality in order to be able to know them thoroughly. By accepting their view and by the understanding that is expressed in this way, clients will gain more trust and are more likely to accept the role division within psychotherapy. It is important that during the first sessions therapists succeed in establishing this role division, consequent expectations and behavioural pattern. The interaction patterns, once established during the first sessions, tend to remain stable in the course of treatment.

With regard to the role division, one may assume that therapists will be recognized by their clients in their role and expert status (Corrigan et al., 1980). Therefore, no status enhancing strategies are usually necessary. What therapists should avoid, however, are behaviour patterns that may lower their status, such as too much self-disclosure (Curtis, 1982).

One must assume that clients may experience some unclarity and hesitation about their own role. No doubt, clients also have specific expectations about psychotherapy. One should, however, question the realism of these expectations. On the other hand, by seeking treatment and by presenting themselves physically to the therapist, they have also evinced a commitment. Together with the legitimate power that clients assign to therapists, this commitment will generate the willingness to accept the definition of the relationship as it is presented by the therapists.

The communication within psychotherapy is targeted mainly towards the person and the behaviour of one person, namely the client. Consequently, speech activity and the extent of self-disclosure are asymmetrically divided. According to the role division within psychotherapy, it is the task of the therapist to establish a particular form of communication that is different from everyday communication. Everyday conventions, such as courtesy and rules of discourse are temporarily suspended. Essential features of the client role are self-responsibility and active participation. Clients should experience their therapists as persons that invest their competent help in the change process. They should at the same time accept that they themselves should contribute actively to the process of change. The therapist functions as a source of stimulation and reinforcement.

With the use of goal-directed explanations and directives, therapists should clarify role expectations. The results of Barkham and Shapiro (1986) show that *instructions* about the expected process of sessions ("process advisement") are experienced by clients as positive and helpful. One may assume that these process advisements will lead to a decrease in clients' uncertainty about their role in psychotherapy. Also, therapists should try to systematically shape this communication style by ignoring or stopping undesirable behaviour and by reinforcing or giving feedback on desirable behaviour. Results from studies on verbal conditioning have shown that the use of explanation and shaping techniques are effective in the generation of particular verbal behaviour such as self-disclosure (Kanfer & Phillips, 1970).

Adoption of the expected role behaviour by clients will be facilitated if they recognize that therapists are being empathic and accepting. It goes without saying that therapists gather information about their clients' life situation. Consequently, with goal-directed *questions* therapists will try to get the most reliable information (Cox, Hopkins & Rutter, 1981). Although clients do not experience such questions as most helpful, they do, however, acknowledge the legitimate need of therapists for information (Elliott et al., 1982b). More information is gathered with open questions than with closed ones (Hill, Carter & O'Farrell, 1983). Asking more than one question at a time should be avoided, as this clearly renders clients uncertain and yields unreliable information. Goal-directed questions about feelings yield most strongly a description of feelings by clients (Hopkinson, Cox & Rutter, 1981).

Expressing *empathy* and paraphrasing or *reflecting* utterances may appear to be a somewhat strange behaviour at times (Wiedemann, 1983). These utterances are, however, experienced by clients as most helpful and generate a feeling of being understood (Elliott, 1979; Elliott, Barker, Caskey & Pistrang, 1982b). In the case that clients express feelings and therapists want the client to explore these, reflections are the most effective utterances for a therapist to use (Hopkinson et al., 1981).

In this opening phase of treatment, therapists should refrain from negative evaluations since these might generate anxiety as a result of their negative associations. This implies that interpretations, as well as confrontations and criticisms, are to be avoided by therapists in this phase of treatment. According to Strong and Claiborn (1982), echoing the clinical intuition of many client-centered therapists, the value-free acceptance of a client's world of experience is the condition *sine qua non* of a client's experience of understanding and trust.

Phase 2: generating the willingness to change

Next for the establishment of a trustful relationship, clients should be induced to expect that change is possible. The situation of clients has been described by Jerome Frank as one of demoralization, i.e. to feel incapable of changing one's situation, characterized by a disbelief to possess the qualities to do so, or ability to employ effectively the necessary behaviour. It is therefore the task of therapists to aid in developing the trust in the clients' skills and outcome and efficacy expectations (Bandura, 1977). This target requires therapists to emphasize and reinforce positive and effective behaviour, i.e. spheres of life that provide clients joy or already successful change attempts. On the basis of concrete events or behaviour, clients may slowly be induced to believe that they do possess the necessary skills to effectuate change.

Support is apparently the best means to achieve this belief. Support comprises all therapist behaviour that reflects positive valuation, as well as encouragement and comforting statements. Several studies have shown that support is experienced positively by clients. It is evaluated as helpful and as empathic (Elliott, Barker, Caskey & Pistrang, 1982a; Elliott, 1986) and is associated with a positive perception of the person of the therapist as well as the session (Ford, 1978; Fuller & Hill, 1985). Obviously, support is also suitable in the development of trust since Snyder, as early as 1945, found that support showed the highest rate of contingent change proposals by the client.

To increase the willingness to change even more, therapists should discuss the advantages and disadvantages of the present situation of the client and design perspectives for a change in the situation. This should also be judged in its positive and negative effects. Therapists should try to look for positive starting points and stimuli for change processes. These interventions represent a first attempt against demoralization and should inform the client about his or her own control over the content and the process of treatment. This motivation for psychotherapy and discussion of strategies to increase this motivation is taken up again in Chapter 3 on problems in psychotherapy.

Phase 3: behavioural analysis

After the establishment of the therapeutic framework during the first sessions, a precise analysis of the problem is conducted, i.e. therapists gather as much information as possible about the symptomatology and the controlling conditions using different diagnostic means. This information is then used to create a behavioural analysis.

In the behavioural analysis, an explanatory model is successively introduced for the problematic behaviours. With goal-directed explanations, the client is invited to participate in this process and in doing so will learn this functional approach. The analysis of a specific problem may generate dissonance when clients are confronted with discrepancies between different behaviour and attitudes (Zimmer, 1983). According to Strong and Matross's model, therapists begin to move away from the clients' frame of reference and lead them in small steps towards their own way of thinking, and looking at problematic situations (Strong & Claiborn, 1982). Accepting the functional way of thinking and looking at problematic behaviour and attitudes, constitutes an important step in this direction.

Next to information gathering, reflection and support, *explanations* are, in the course of the behavioural analysis, important interventions. Elliott (1986) reported that explanations were judged by clients to be one of the most helpful classes of therapist behaviour. Problem descriptions seem to occur most often contingently with explanations (Hill et al., 1983; Hochdörfer, Ludwig, Rhenius & Lasgoga, 1983). This finding may be interpreted as the acceptance of the explanation by clients when they clarify the explained state of affairs by use of examples from their own life.

Interpretation is another important verbal therapist behaviour during the behavioural analysis. In the behavioural therapeutic context this should be perceived as the description of a state of affairs in terms of learning theoretical terms. Although the impact of interpretation seems to be somewhat contradictory, as previously defined, interpretations seem helpful in that they clarify the translation of the functional thinking in regard to the clients' situation.

Phase 4: the treatment program

At the closure of the behavioural analysis, therapists, on the basis of the information available, construct a preliminary conditional model. Using this model they can explain to their clients the origin and the controlling factors of their problems. For the further course of treatment it is absolutely necessary that this model is tailored to the individual clients, considered plausible and, at least in principle, accepted by them. It should describe their central problems and clarify the connections between the origin, the controlling factors, and the possible changes regarding experiences and behaviour (Reinecker, 1987). From this functional model, targets and therapeutic interventions are deduced. If clients accept this model, an important step in the increase of cognitive dissonance has occurred, since the model implies the possibility of change. This dissonance can only be reduced by changes in the problematic behaviour and attitudes.

Phase 5: conducting the treatment

With the conduction of the planned therapy, therapists introduce successive proposals and techniques of change. They have to take care, however, that the different steps fall within the tolerance level of clients. On the other hand, the steps should not be too difficult and require too much cost for the client. The successful victory over a small task enhances the probability of embarking on a much more difficult task later (Freedman & Fraser, 1966).

This phase is characterized by *advice* and other directives by therapists. Clear directives are expected by clients (e.g. Reid & Shapiro, 1969) and experienced as helpful (Elliott et al., 1982b; Elliott, 1986). Whereas advisements during the first sessions are experienced negatively, later on in therapy they become inevitable and necessary.

A decrease in empathic statements is observed in this phase of treatment (Gustavson, Jansson, Jerremalm & Öst, 1985). Although reflective statements tend to generate trust in the beginning of treatment, they also constitute reinforcements and may under certain circumstances prevent attitude changes (Johnson & Matross, 1977).

Disturbing influences and failures should be recognized by therapists at the right time. They may consist of dropout, noncompliance and resistance. Behaviour therapists have originally been oriented towards preventing resistance. In support of this clinical intuition is the finding that therapists with a high rate of support were associated with low rates of resistance amongst their clients. Nevertheless, if resistance in whatever form occurs, a rational solution of the problem is advised (Caspar & Grawe, 1981). Elsewhere strategies are suggested to handle resistance on a communicational level (Zimmer, 1983). Strategies such as "paradoxical prescription" and the "offer of false alternatives" have been described. Regarding the latter method, the client is provided with a choice in the "how" of the conduction of a particular assignment or intervention, while at the same time no doubt will be possible about the actual conduction of the task. We will describe more extensively examples of such strategic procedures in Part II. Although these formulations are derived well from social psychological theories, the empirical test of their effectiveness is still lacking (Shoham-Salomon & Rosenthal, 1987).

Phase 6: monitoring and evaluating progress

In each stage of learning, clients have to be sensitized to progress towards the therapeutic goals. Therapists should consequently assess and provide feedback on any positive change. In other words, support by the therapist is of extreme importance. On the one hand, support implies positive feedback, recognition for changes achieved, and an approach towards the therapeutic goal. On the other hand, a capacity for change is demonstrated which provides encouragement for further attempts. Barkham and Shapiro (1986) report that support during the fourth session is as likely as reflection to lead to understanding and insight. Important in this phase is also *confrontation*. Frank and Sweetland (1962) and Hill et al. (1983) report an increased contingency of *insight* after confrontation.

Phase 7: generalizing the progress and the dissolution of the bond

The (external) control by the therapist over the client is slowly reduced until the point in time that therapeutic contact becomes superfluous. The behaviour of therapists will at the closure of therapy contain less directives and more support. The self-help skills that clients have developed during treatment should be reinforced. Special attention should be given to relapse prevention, to the identification of situations with a high probability of relapsing into the problematic behaviour and attitudes. Therapy will be terminated when clients feel secure and able to handle problems themselves, eventually together with their spouses and other persons in their social environment. According to Strong and Claiborn (1982), therapists have then succeeded in leading their clients into a new system of relationships. There is no more need for the client to use the resources of the therapist. Consequently, the relationship may be dissolved.

Evaluation of the process model

With the introduction of social psychological principles in behavioural psychotherapy, a theoretical framework becomes available that enables the description and explanation of social aspects of therapy as well as an operationalization of related constructs. This theoretical framework cannot be considered complete, however. One reason is that the social psychological model itself contains many problems (see Heppner & Claiborn, 1989). As already pointed out, most studies are analogue in nature and comparable to an interview or a first therapeutic session. Although we do not question the value of analogue research (Kazdin, 1986), more studies are needed that take into account the process feature of psychotherapy. Another problem is the fact that the model is incomplete. For instance, crisis intervention is not included in the first phase. Many therapeutic interventions are geared to dealing with crises by structural changes, e.g. within a family system.

This social psychological model, however, seems particularly useful to fill a theoretical gap in the concept of therapeutic change. The described theses are useful in explaining the impact of the psychotherapeutic relationship on the client. Change takes place within clients, and the social interaction within psychotherapy provides the conditions for the consequent learning processes. To explain the ensuing changes, behavioural theory is well equipped.

The next step should consist of the operationalization of further strategies of social influence. This means that the social psychological framework has to be filled with empirically founded advisements for therapists on how to handle particular clients, i.e. which concrete behaviour will succeed in motivating this client to make the investments necessary for reaching the subgoals in each phase. In other words, how can therapists generate trust in clients, motivate them to participate actively and generate a working alliance? Kanfer and Grimm (1980) and Kanfer et al. (1990) provided the first hypotheses with the formulation of their model.

In the next three chapters more clinically derived strategies will be presented that do, however, need further empirical testing.

Part II
CLINICAL IMPLICATIONS: STRATEGIES FOR MANAGING THE THERAPEUTIC RELATIONSHIP

Part II is devoted to the management of the therapeutic relationship in behavioural psychotherapy. The section begins with Chapter 3, in which three important problems in the therapeutic relationship are presented: dropout, noncompliance and reactance. The literature is summarized and a model of motivation strategies, developed on the basis of an extensive literature review, is presented, fitting well with the process model described in chapter 2. In Chapters 4 and 5, we describe the strategies to engage patients in therapy and strategies to maintain a collaborative set.

3 Problems in clinical practice: dropout, noncompliance and reactance

Introduction

In the following section, we challenge the long-cherished proposition that clients must adapt to the therapists' psychotherapeutic style in order for behavioural change to occur. Change is more likely to occur if therapists adapt to the way clients view their role in the change process and present themselves. We demonstrate how therapists can change their behaviour in ways that enable clients to experience the relationship more positively, to participate actively, and thereby succeed in treatment goals.

It is surprising that few psychotherapeutic schools pay explicitly attention to the "client-is-king" position. Most handbooks of psychotherapy focus exclusively on technical issues, with the exception of the interactional and paradoxical approach, as was shown in an analysis of the literature used for training therapists in different schools of psychotherapy in the Netherlands (Bekkers & Schaap, 1985).

Part I of this volume is devoted to the theoretical conceptualization of the therapeutic relationship in behavioural psychotherapy. This chapter will present concrete case studies from clinical practice, which relate to different phases of the process model presented in Chapter 2. The case descriptions represent typical problems in the process of psychotherapy related to the client-therapist relationship and transcend the mere application of therapeutic techniques. Emphasis is placed upon the formulation of strategies that represent solutions for problematic situations in engaging the client and in maintaining a collaborative set.

We will first describe the following problems in clinical practice: dropout, noncompliance and reactance. We will then describe strategies for coping with these problems that are derived from three sources: motivation for psychotherapy, the interpersonal style of the client and the quality of the therapeutic relationship.

The phase model described in the preceding chapter highlights a number of problems that may occur in the relationship between client and therapist. Some of these problems are related to specific phases in the therapeutic process. The first issue in the effective implementation of a treatment programme is to successfully *engage* potential clients. It is a well established fact that exposure is an effective technique in the treatment of anxiety disorders. Despite this fact, many clients who are referred for treatment *refuse* to participate. Since this issue is not a problem related to the therapeutic relationship itself, but rather to marketing and public relations, it will not be focused on in this section.

The second problem in clinical practice is clients *dropping out* of treatment. Here we speak of motivating the client, once engaged in therapy, to participate actively in the therapeutic process. The third problem is lack of active cooperation or *reactance* on the part of the client. As will be clear from the discussion in the preceding chapter, the latter term is preferred since it denotes a social psychological phenomenon referring to a process of self-protection in response to the therapist "intruding" into an area of personal freedom for the client. In a medical context this process is referred to as "noncompliance with medical advice". We will present strategies on how to cope with this issue in treatment. The final problem highlighted by the process model is *relapse*. Relapse implies that, following a more or less symptom-free phase, a worsening of symptoms occurs. In the case of a good therapeutic relationship, relapse would probably lead to the patient seeing the therapist again. So in some cases a good relationship would prevent a lengthy relapse of symptoms. Nevertheless, since relapse is not necessarily a problem of the therapeutic relationship, but rather the result of a neglect on the part of the therapist to focus on coping with high-risk situations, we will not address it further in this chapter.

We will describe three sources in the treatment process for choosing strategies to handle the above problems. These sources are labeled motivation for psychotherapy, the interpersonal style of the client and the quality of the therapeutic relationship. It is interesting that these sources are available to therapists to a differing extent in the initial phases of the therapeutic process.

Some information about the extent to which the client is *motivated* to participate actively in treatment is usually available to therapists before any contact has taken place. The manner in which the client is referred to the therapist as well as his or her level of complaints are particularly helpful in deducing the client's motivation for seeking help. In addition, it is also possible to further assess the motivation on the part of the client with the aid of a variety of instruments. Literature on this will be presented in this chapter.

Once a contact has been established, be it by phone, letter or person-to-person contact, some conclusions can be drawn about the *interpersonal style* of the client, in terms of the social psychological dimensions of affiliation and dominance. These conclusions may be further validated and tested by the therapist over the course of treatment, again using different instruments and methods. More concretely, we will describe motivating strategies for handling domineering, paranoid, obstructive, complaining and dependent clients.

Finally, after two or three sessions, clients and therapists can reliably assess the *quality of their relationship*. This constitutes the third source for deriving strategies to motivate clients and to handle interpersonal problems in treatment. The choice of any of these strategies may be based on the scores of clients and therapists on instruments measuring the relationship, i.e., the way the participants view each other.

We will now present a case illustrating the problems of dropout and reactance, as well as some solutions for coping with these problems.

A case description

Mr Jones is a 35-year-old man who has suffered from compulsive symptoms and obsessional ruminations for approximately 10 years. He spends numerous hours each day meticulously inspecting his face for any skin irregularities, such as loose skin and acne. If he discovers such horrors, he mercilessly squeezes and scratches his face to remove their presence. Consequently, his face is pock-marked with small scars. He is extremely self-conscious about these scars and thus avoids meeting other people or going out. He is unemployed and lives from a government allowance. These problems seriously affect his marriage, and his wife is left to do all the shopping and household chores. If he is not inspecting his face, Mr Jones remains in bed during the day, and then is more active in the evenings. He goes to bed long after his wife; as a result the couple's sexual relationship has suffered. Apart from going to classes twice a week, Mr Jones has seemingly given up all other outside interests.

Mr Jones has not asked for his wife to assist him with this compulsive rituals, nor has he sought reassurance from her, even though it is impossible for him to follow through any plans that they make together. For example, if they decide to go to the cinema or go out and visit relatives, he will suddenly start inspecting and scratching his skin, and if they succeed in going anywhere at all, they are always late. Mrs Jones is a friendly, yet somewhat insecure woman who shows doubt about being able to keep up this lifestyle, even though she is prepared continually to sacrifice herself. Mr Jones has previously received several years of outpatient treatment from a psychiatric social service agency, but this did not produce any noticeable improvement. His obsessive thoughts result in increased tension, which he relieves by scratching his skin.

After the first assessment session, further treatment was offered to both partners. A 10 session treatment contract was agreed upon, after which an evaluation would take place and a decision made about continuation. If no improvement occurred by the 10th session, it would be assumed that this method of treatment was not appropriate and a referral to another agency would then be arranged.

In looking at some of the processes of treatment and the eventual outcome, Mr Jones requests help initially for his compulsive scratching. The therapist agrees and discusses the need for detailed assessment. He is given a clock of the type that is used by chess players which indicates the time that is left for a move. In this way, he monitors his scratching on the left clock and the time he is showing appropriate non-scratching behaviour on the right clock. Before scratching, he starts the chess clock and, when finished, he has to push the button engaging the other clock. Care is taken in thoroughly explaining the therapeutic procedure of exposure and response prevention in order to motivate Mr Jones to carry out the self-monitoring task.

At the following session, Mr Jones admits that he was unable to monitor his scratching; he reports that he forgot, placing the therapist in an awkward position. The therapist is confronted either with a motivational problem or was perhaps not successful in explaining the rationale of the assignment. Again the therapist explains the importance of monitoring as a first step in overcoming the compulsive behaviour and the task is repeated. Following this session, Mr Jones reports successfully monitoring for a few days, indicating that a start had been achieved. The therapist then formulates this as follows: "Apparently, you are so involved in your compulsive behaviour that you are unable to monitor it". He then asks Mrs Jones if she would pay attention to when her husband scratches his face. She agrees to manage the chess clock during the time that she is at home.

At the fourth session, it is clear that Mr Jones is able to monitor his behaviour himself and the treatment then proceeds by compiling an inventory of all activities he is unable to do. To prevent any deterioration in the relationship and to provide support for Mr Jones, the therapist discusses the importance of joint activities. It is further explained that the aim of treatment is to allow him to continue scratching his face, but that each time, attempts will be made to make it more difficult for him to do so. Treatment proceeds with the application of behaviour therapy with exposure and response prevention until the eighth session. The couple arrive late following an argument about the monitoring, which again they had discontinued. The arguments are then discussed during the session and are prescribed in a more positive context, as a sign that they care a great deal about each other. Again, the need for assessing the scratching is emphasized. At the beginning of the 10th session, Mr Jones with a triumphant smile, puts the chess clock on the therapist's desk declaring that he has decided to discontinue the treatment and is then referred to another agency.

In terms of a DSM-III-R (American Psychiatric Association 1987) diagnosis, Mr Jones presents an anxiety disorder, more specifically an obsessive–compulsive disorder (Axis I) with accompanying marital problems (Axis III) and is unable to maintain a job (Axis V). The therapist proposed time-limited therapy as a way of encouraging him to comply, while accepting that neither the client or therapist would be responsible if the treatment prove to be unsuccessful. In the event of the treatment not being successful, it could then be assumed that it was not the right approach for his problem. Finally, in case of failure, re-referral would be possible so the couple would not drop out of the care system completely.

Upon reviewing this case, we note that the patient was treated with the specific techniques of exposure and response prevention, a behavioural treatment method applied successfully for obsessive-compulsive symptoms (Emmelkamp, 1982). He was progressively exposed to the anxiety-provoking thoughts and situations, a penalty for exhibiting more responses than was agreed upon was introduced. The penalty consisted of doing unpleasant, but necessary household chores and activities that neutralized his social isolation, or doing interesting or even pleasant activities that could easily be postponed (e.g., attending a course or working on a hobby).

During Mr Jones' treatment programmeme, it was necessary to assess his compulsive behaviours and obsessive thoughts. To do this successfully, the therapist first *explained* the rationale of treatment and *emphasized* the need for reliable monitoring. After the first report of failure, the therapist again explained the rationale of the treatment procedure by pointing out its importance. When in the next session it appeared that there were difficulties with the task, the therapist interpreted the behaviour as a sign of reactance, a motivational problem, or even a struggle for power in the therapeutic relationship. Whichever it was, the therapist *labeled* the problematic behaviour positively for the patient and his spouse, by saying that the patient was apparently so absorbed in his compulsive behaviour or that the compulsive behaviour was so overwhelming that he was unable to monitor it. The *pressure* was increased and the reactance was *utilised* by involving the spouse in the home assignment. Initially, this produces a positive result, so the next phase of treatment could commence. The average time the patient scratched his face was calculated and a target time during which the patient was allowed to scratch without "punishment" was negotiated. Failure to achieve the target on a particular day was "paid for" by doing something useful, in this case some household chores. At the point that relaxation training was introduced, the couple's marital problems become more overt.

During the eighth and ninth session reactance again emerged and the couple argued because of their miserable lifestyle, which was determined by the compulsive problems which, in fact, had begun to change. By exposing the marital problem, a power struggle with the therapist ensued and again, monitoring became a problem. By labeling the arguments positively, as a means of showing that they cared about each other, the therapist succeeded in creating some stability and was able to deal with the reactance. Again, the assignment was explained to the couple, but this time it was unsuccessful. The patient's triumphant gesture when returning the chess clock indicates that he felt that he had achieved a measure of victory over the therapist. It is important to note that during the entire treatment period of 10 weeks, the therapist tried to be *empathic* and *courteous* towards the patient.

This case illustrates some of the common problems that occur in treatment. At the same time, it illustrates some of the strategies and techniques therapists may use to foster the therapeutic relationship and motivate clients to comply with particular therapeutic procedures. In the following section, we will attempt to describe some of these problems and some of the solutions that have been suggested in the literature. In many cases, with these strategies, therapists can overcome the problems of dropout, noncompliance and reactance. However, as was the case with Mr Jones, these strategies will not always result in a positive outcome or even be successful in keeping the client in treatment. We hope with these strategies, to provide the therapist some room to manoeuvre, leading to success in overcoming problematic episodes in treatment and sometimes in a "sleeper" effect, i.e., result in a positive outcome in later treatment.

Problems in clinical practice

Dropout

Dropout appears to have a variety of definitions, presenting a considerable methodological problem. It is often defined in terms of duration of treatment: someone is labeled a dropout if he or she has not followed a pre-set number of sessions. The criterion of classification is sometimes arbitrary, often on the basis of the median number of sessions (Baekeland & Lundwall, 1975). This is problematic, since in most studies a different number of sessions is used as the criterion for classifying dropouts. Additionally, there is no relationship between the duration of treatment and dropout.

There are a number of other definitions that have been used and reported in the literature. These include having outcome evaluations from both participants that fall below the mean number of sessions (Tracey, 1986), being in need of continued treatment beyond the last session (Pekarik, 1983), a view of the therapist that treatment is in the initial stage, in progress or incomplete (Garfield, 1986), before the therapeutic process has been completed (Walrond-Skinner, 1986), when the treatment goals agreed upon by both the therapist and client have not been achieved, and when the therapist believes that additional sessions are essential and indeed will result in further improvement (Emmelkamp & Foa, 1983). A definition that is conceptually more appropriate views the dropout as the person who has unilaterally withdrawn from therapy at some point, either explicitly against the advice of the therapist or implicitly, cancelling appointments and failing to recontract (Cross & Warren, 1984).

Obviously the ideal moment of ending psychotherapy will depend on the method of treatment and the therapist's theoretical framework. The extent to which treatment goals have been agreed upon will facilitate this decision considerably, especially in time-limited forms of psychotherapy, such as behavioural and cognitive psychotherapy.

Baekeland and Lundwall (1975) reviewed the clinical literature on treatment dropout, in which they included studies on psychiatric treatment, the treatment of tuberculosis, high blood pressure, pharmacological treatment and substance abuse. They reported that the prevalence of dropout after the first session in a psychiatric clinic ranges from 20 to 57%. Similar figures are presented for group psychotherapy, and 32 to 79% of clinic patients in open psychiatric wards discontinue their treatment after the first few months. Higher figures are reported for patients presenting substance abuse; 50 to 75% of clients in outpatient alcohol and heroine treatment programmemes do not return after their fourth appointment. Relatively high dropout figures are also reported for clients suffering from essential hypertension, most probably because they do not experience adverse symptoms.

It is interesting to take a look at the literature supporting dropout as related to factors in the client-therapist relationship. Baekeland and Lundwall (1975) identified a number of factors that determined dropout, some of which related to the client-therapist relationship. They found that clients from lower socio-economic classes are more likely to drop out of treatment, suggesting that this may reflect the inconsistency between their expectations and values and those of therapists. Furthermore, socially isolated people were found to be more likely to discontinue treatment probably because of lack of support or an inability to attach themselves to others including the therapist. Other factors that were identified included social instability, symptom levels and symptom relief, aggression and motivation for psychotherapy.

Greenspan and Kulish (1985) found the following factors to differentiate between those who continued and those who dropped out of therapy: age, race, referral source, employment status, type of payment, complaint and diagnosis. They describe the likely treatment terminator to be a "young well paid black worker" referred for therapy from another clinical setting.

It was found that counsellor–client agreement on the nature of the problem was the single most important factor determining continuing in treatment. McNair, Lorr and Callahan (1963) found those who remain in treatment to have a history of less impulsivity, less anti-social behaviour, admitting to more anxious behaviour, being more self-critical and less likely to endorse irrational beliefs.

Fiester and Rudestan (1975) argue that dropout phenomena may reflect therapeutic factors that at first appear to be counter-intuitive. They give the example of some clients wanting treatment to facilitate an authoritarian battle and, if this does not occur, they discontinue their treatment.

According to Baekeland and Lundwall (1975), the phenomenon of dropout is the result of three sets of variables: intrapsychic client factors (demographic, clinical, personality); therapist variables (personality, attitude to the client and style of therapy); and environmental variables (cost of treatment, attitude of the family, transport). The authors believe that dropouts consist of three particular types of clients, including those who do not succeed in returning to treatment, those who refuse to return and those who are removed from treatment. There also appear to be critical stages in the duration of treatment that indicate dropout; after one (intake) session, after 1 month and between the second and sixth month.

Phillips (1985) presented the results of a number of literature reviews and empirical studies on clients discontinuing treatment, which he referred to as *attrition*. He showed that if the data that are reported in studies on number of sessions and clients remaining in treatment at each session were presented graphically, the result is a negatively accelerating Poisson distribution, regardless of the type of institution or treatment. Phillips noted that studies of dropout have almost exclusively focused on client demographic variables and that they have failed to find robust relationships. It seems most likely that the decision to remain in treatment depends on the way that the therapeutic situation fulfils the needs and perceptions of the client and the way the healthcare system operates.

There are a few studies reporting data on clients' reasons for dropout. Garfield, Affleck & Muffly (1963) interviewed 24 outpatients about their reasons for terminating treatment. The diagnoses varied and included neurosis, character or personality disturbance and psychosis and a quantitative criterion, i.e., attending for less than seven sessions. Of this group of 24 clients, 12 met this criterion and of these 12, 11 were traced and interviewed. Six identified external circumstances which made it impossible to continue with treatment (transport, childcare, work) three indicated dissatisfaction with their therapist and only two reported having stopped therapy because they felt sufficiently improved. Compared with the other group of 12 clients who received seven sessions or more, external factors were reported more often by the 11 dropouts as a reason to stop treatment.

Acosta (1980) defined dropouts as those who ended therapy within six sessions without consulting the therapist. The 74 patients from three ethnic groups, again having varying diagnoses, were contacted by telephone. Most of these clients indicated dissatisfaction with their therapist or problems in the therapeutic relationship or the mode of treatment; only 20% indicated improvement. In this study, external factors were also mentioned as reasons for dropout.

Pekarik (1983) defined a dropout as a client who withdrew from treatment against therapeutic advice. Forty-six dropouts were interviewed by telephone about their reasons for discontinuing treatment. Approximately half indicated dissatisfaction with the help they received and 25% indicated dissatisfaction with the therapist. Pekarik pointed out that external factors are sometimes used by clients to avoid criticizing the treatment they received. Furthermore, he stated that the often reported practical problems may be indicative of low motivation.

Emmelkamp and Van der Hout (1983) sent a questionnaire to 15 agoraphobics who dropped out of treatment. Half of the clients who returned the questionnaire identified problems in the therapeutic relationship as reasons for their withdrawal. A pilot study in an outpatient centre on a sample of five clients suffering from anxiety disorders (Jessen, 1989) revealed comparable figures. Similar percentages were reported by Hansen, Hoogduin, Schaap and de Haan (1992) in their follow-up study of obsessive-compulsive patients. In this latter study it was found that dropouts differed from a matched successful control group in that the latter experienced significantly more pressure from a spouse or family member to seek or to remain in treatment. This is an interesting phenomenon, even if it may apply only to obsessive-compulsive patients.

These studies all show that dropout is a major problem in delivering mental health care. We must assume that a percentage of dropouts can be accounted for by their perceived problems in the therapeutic relationship. When external factors are reported as reasons for not continuing, low initial motivation may be indicated, or perhaps experienced problems in the therapeutic relationship were not disclosed earlier. It is clear from the above that the therapeutic relationship can be used as a vehicle to improve motivation and to reduce dropout or attrition. Further research in this neglected area is essential. Enhancing a strong therapeutic relationship in an early phase of treatment could possibly prevent dropout in some cases.

Reactance and noncompliance

Clients often seek treatment not necessarily because they want solutions for their problems but as a result of the negative consequences of their problematic behaviour. Low self-esteem, social isolation, reduction in the quality of their close relationships, or loss of time, money, a job or health are the reasons often given for seeking help, rather than problematic behaviour itself. Phobias and rituals may be functional in that they are used as a way of dealing with anxiety and stress. Even when the symptoms are a sign of having lost control over one's life, we as therapists experience *reactance*, noncompliance and lack of co-operation from clients with given treatment directives. Further, changes in existing behavioural patterns lead to feelings of discomfort, anxiety and depression which can lead to reactance as well. Many authors have tried to study resistance/reactance and have developed methods of measuring it.

Watzlawick, Beavin, and Jackson (1967) described resistant interviewees' behaviour characteristically as directly expressing opinions through refusing to co-operate, but there are other indirect ways of expressing this unwillingness. This can be expressed by keeping the conversation superficial, by disqualifications, inconsistencies and contradictions in the narrative, unfinished sentences, and vague use of language, mannerisms and affected speech.

The term *compliance* is used in medicine to refer to the extent that the patient follows the physician's directives. Research shows that characteristics inherent in the doctor–patient interaction are important determinants of noncompliance (Becker & Mainman, 1980). Factors within the therapeutic relationship that have been found to be associated with patient's failure to comply with advice and directives include instances when therapists show complete disagreement with the patient's opinions, where the therapist is rejecting, too formal and controlling, and where the patient's expectations have not been fulfilled. Other variables associated with the conduct of treatment may also influence compliance; for example, the earlier the task is assigned in the treatment contract, the greater is the likelihood of compliance.

Although the concept of noncompliance, as used in medicine, is somewhat problematic in psychotherapy, the implications are quite clear. Noncompliance is comparable to unco-operative behaviour, inhibiting behaviour, reactance, resistance and non-accommodation with the therapeutic regime. As already stated, change and personal development are not without pain and difficulty, but are characterized rather by friction, difficulties and dislike. Reactance can manifest itself within and outside the treatment situation as well as in extra-therapeutic events (coming late, missing appointments, not paying, asking for favours, giving presents) and, eventually, it may result in the complete discontinuation of treatment, i.e., dropout. Outside of the session, reactance may be expressed through refusing or only partly completing therapeutic assignments. During the session, it can become manifest through a refusal to talk about specific topics, talking about trivialities or avoiding eye contact.

Resistant behaviour, labeled as reactance or noncompliance, opposes positive outcome and attempts are usually made to overcome it. However, it is important to raise the question, is it really such a negative event? Should it be identified and opposed at all costs? A number of studies indicate that the presence of reactance in certain phases of treatment is associated with positive outcome. Orlinsky and Howard (1978), following an extensive review of relevant studies from different psychotherapeutic schools, suggested that reactance in the middle phase of treatment can be associated with positive outcome. A similar trend was found in the study of self-control procedures in a group of problem drinkers (Schaap & Schippers, 1985). It is possible therefore that these behaviours could also be considered as signs of responsiveness. This is consistent with those forms of psychotherapy using paradoxical interventions which encourage reactance, as will be illustrated at a later point (Tennen et al., 1981).

In the following pages we will try to describe in more detail three sources that determine the effectiveness of using strategies to motivate clients to change. These three sources are: (a) motivation for psychotherapy, (b) the interpersonal style of the client (and the therapist), and (c) the quality of the therapeutic relationship. Each of these sources will yield a number of strategies that may be used in clinical practice to deal with the problems of dropout, noncompliance and reactance.

Therapist flexibility in relation to clients: developing motivational strategies

Motivation for psychotherapy

Although the notion of motivation for psychotherapy is not well understood, it is nevertheless important in a discussion of problems in psychotherapy. The factors (to be presented later in this chapter) that are considered in the literature to be indicative of motivation for psychotherapy are heterogeneous and varied and, more often than not, have been formulated on the basis of interviews with psychotherapists. These factors have then been related to therapy outcome and it is on the basis of these data that relevant questionnaires have been constructed. The scores on such questionnaires appear to be related to outcome (which is not surprising) and are then used to indicate which patients are suitable for a certain form of psychotherapy.

This somewhat overcharged picture demonstrates that, more often than not, motivation for psychotherapy is used as a means to select clients for psychotherapy. As already pointed out, this way of working is not ideal from our point of view. Measuring motivation for psychotherapy should be used as a source for selecting interpersonal strategies that will increase the probability that a client will engage in therapy, will remain in treatment and will actively cooperate with the therapist. In the end, this should lead to a lessening of symptomatology and to an attitude change (Frank, 1973). We will present the pertinent literature here in somewhat more detail.

Dean (1958) proposed that clients can be placed on a behavioural continuum at the start of therapy. The stages of the continuum included open animosity, negativism, passive resistance, neutrality and accepting psychological problems. Mr Jones, the case described earlier, would probably be rated as a passive resistant. His attitude to therapy, expressed by the problems with the monitoring assignment, was at best ambivalent.

The following constructs are reported in the literature to be indicative of motivation for psychotherapy (Appelbaum, 1972; Badura, 1975, 1976; Dean, 1958; Engel & Wilms, 1986; Keithley, 1985; Kernberg et al., 1972; Krause, 1964, 1966, 1967, 1968; Rosenbaum & Horowitz, 1983; Schwab & Mathieson, 1979; Siegel & Fink, 1962; Sifneos, 1971, 1975; Weber, 1984):

- extent of suffering,
- recognizing the existence of a psychological problem,
- the desire for change,
- own initiative in seeking treatment (versus being sent),
- being prepared to make sacrifices,
- internal locus of control,
- accepting the client role,
- recognizing the problem as psychological (versus somatic),
- introspective capability,
- honesty,
- realistic expectations,
- active participation,
- secondary gains,
- openness,
- curiosity or need to understand oneself,
- interpersonal attraction,
- earlier experiences with psychotherapy,
- self-confidence,
- the value attached to psychotherapy,
- demographic variables,
- tolerance of stigmatization,
- frustration tolerance,
- opinion of (significant) others about the problem.

On the basis of this literature Kersten, Hoogduin and Schaap (1988) developed the Nijmegen Motivation List (NML), a self-report questionnaire to be rated by the client and intended to measure different aspects of motivation for psychotherapy. The NML consists of the following items:

1   My complaints make me feel very unhappy.
2   In spite of my complaints I can function well in daily life.
3   I am prepared to do anything in order to overcome my complaints.
4   Because of my complaints, I am unable to fulfill a number of necessary responsibilities.
5   Because of my complaints people are more considerate than usual towards me.
6   I entered therapy on the advice of others.
7   I expect that therapy will do me more good if I invest myself actively in it.
8   Whatever happens, I will carry out therapeutic tasks.
9   I have little confidence in the outcome of the proposed therapy.

10 I think that my complaints have a somatic origin.
11 The cause of my complaints reflect my circumstances.
12 I am known to be persistent.

Keijsers, Schaap and Hoogduin (1990) gave the NML to 53 clients presenting with anxiety disorders, before their intake session, i.e., before any personal contact between the client and intaker or therapist had been made. To
measure outcome of treatment, the Symptom Checklist (SCL-90; Arrindell &
Ettema, 1986; Derogatis, 1977) was used before the first and last session.
Factor analysis on the scores of the NML yielded two factors: (1) extent of
suffering and (2) belief in the treatment. The variance explained by these factors was moderate (26%), as was the correlation between these two factors
with outcome ($r = 0.28$). Using regression analysis, the results indicated that
the items measuring the extent of suffering and disability caused by the
symptoms (items no. 2 and 4) showed a significant positive correlation with outcome.

Though these results still need be replicated in other studies and in other settings, the items of the NML together can be thought of as a prognostic indicator. Therapists could try to motivate the clients who have (relatively) low
scores on the relevant items. The authors suggest that treatment should not
begin until clients show positive scores, thereby reducing the risk of dropout,
noncompliance and reactance.

Kanfer and Schefft (1988) considered motivation for psychotherapy to be a
need to change, resulting from an imbalance between an actual situation and a
desired state of affairs. According to these authors the question should not
be: Is there motivation for psychotherapy? But rather: How strong is the
desire for a specific change? The sequence of change therefore is: a situation
characterized by suffering, dissonance and imbalance, followed by a particular (sequence of) action (i.e., therapeutic procedures and influence strategies)
that will lead to a desired situation (satisfaction, balance, decrease in level of
complaint). In such a model, motivation for psychotherapy implies utterances by clients that represent their desire for change or an agreement with
particular assignments. And this equals commitment (see also Miller, 1985,
for related literature on addiction).

This very simple model immediately leads to a number of strategies that may
be derived out of the three phases: (a) the actual situation, (b) the desired
state and (c) actions that lead to change.

Effective strategies focusing on the actual situation are, as suggested by these
authors:

● emphasizing the negative consequences of the actual situation,
● giving a monitoring assignment that will lead to breaking the chain of
  habit behaviour,

- changing the criteria for self-monitoring,
- changing deficits in particular skills by role playing,
- changing attributions,
- presenting new information.

Effective strategies focusing on the desired state of affairs are:

- emphasizing the positive consequences of this new state,
- fantasizing about this new state,
- emphasizing positive experiences with this desired state in the past,
- using role playing to create the experience of the positive consequences,
- offering an appropriate coping model.

Effective strategies focusing on the actions that will lead to the desired state are:

- developing a sense of self-efficacy by support and experiences of success,
- setting realistic goals,
- setting subgoals,
- emphasizing responsibility for therapy procedures and success,
- giving assignments that guarantee success,
- to the extent that a good therapeutic relationship is established, making use of paradoxes and provocation,
- working through resistance by exploration, reflection and confrontation.

In the following sections we will develop the suggestions of Kanfer and Schefft more extensively in the context of the next two sources for strategies in coping with problematic situations in treatment: the interpersonal style of the client and the quality of the therapeutic relationship.

The interpersonal style of the client

Harry Stack Sullivan was one of the first authors to recognize the important role of interaction and communication in the etiology and treatment of a variety of psychopathological disorders. He noted that people tend to develop a characteristic way of interacting with others (*interaction style*). This interaction style can be seen more clearly to the extent that it is less varied, more consistent and more extreme. Interaction styles contain more or less hidden appeals by way of which the behaviour of persons is directed (Beier, 1966; Kiesler, 1982; Leary, 1957; Sullivan, 1953). In order to define the characteristics of interaction styles that lead to problems in treatment, Keijsers et al. (1990) analysed the clinical literature in which problems in motivation for psychotherapy were described in the context of personality characteristics of clients. These authors found support for their contention that problems in motivation are often mentioned in connection with a rigid and extreme style of interaction. The analyses of these interactions styles led to the formulation of five "difficult" types of clients: domineering, paranoid, obstructive, complaining and dependent. These types can be related to existing categorizations (Kiesler, 1983; Leary, 1957; APA, 1987). We also encountered strategies on how to handle these clients.

The domineering client   These clients, also labeled self-assured, dominant, competitive (Kiesler, 1983) and bossy–autocratic (Leary, 1957), share features of the narcissistic and obsessive-compulsive personality disorders as distinguished in DSM-III-R (APA, 1987). They are characterized by their self-assured, determining and coercive way of interacting with other people. They are experienced as independent and energetic, and are appealing to a certain degree to other people. To motivate these clients for psychotherapy, they have to be handled in a courteous and respectful manner. They may experience problems in taking on the client role, in their dependent position in therapy and in the doings of therapists. The therapist should therefore be modest and should certainly not imply that he or she perceives things better than does the client. Therapists have to listen interestedly, to advise sparingly and to respect the way the client has managed thus far. Proposals for change and assignments should be presented in such a way that the client can always make a choice (Tennen et al, 1981).

The paranoid client   These clients, also labeled cold and distrustful (Kiesler, 1983), share features of the paranoid and anti-social personality disorders as distinguished by DSM-III-R (APA, 1987). They experience the world as threatening and hostile. The sincerity, loyalty and faith of other people is easily doubted. They take good care not to be used by other people and are serious, critical, reserved and defensive. As a consequence they need be handled correctly and with care. Their self-contentment, prejudice and criticism may raise irritation. And the therapist without self-control will confirm all the negative things that the client expected (Millon, 1981). The therapist needs to be courteous, attentive and tolerant, without submission or capitulation or an air of authority and prestige (Millon, 1981). The therapist should be relaxed, careful in word choice and should not speak for too long (Tennen et al., 1981). Moralizing and personal points of view are taboo. The focus is on actual and observable behaviours and events (McGuire, 1985). To achieve something with paranoid clients, therapists have to use indirect ways and suggestions and have to accept the paranoid world of their clients. If these clients have to be convinced, this has to be achieved by giving careful and factual information with much clarity.

The obstructive client   These clients, also labeled hostile and uninvolved (Kiesler, 1983) and rebellious–distrustful (Leary, 1957), share features of the following personality disorders distinguished by DSM-III-R (APA, 1987):

passive–aggressive, anti-social, schizotypical and borderline. They experience serious problems in conforming to social norms, in relational expectations and in their professional duties. They are experienced as unpredictable, obstructive and explosive and, in this way, create considerable personal distance. They often feel a lack of appreciation, seem continually disappointed in other people, are cynical and have low self-esteem. Opposition may be expressed openly or, more often than not, in a pattern of continuous forgetting and postponement. Such clients may eventually bring the therapist to his or her end. However, what this client needs is a friendly, patient and courteous approach as is affirmed by clinical authors (Millon, 1981; Van der Velden, 1985). Therapists should remain friendly, interested and tolerant. Whenever clients criticize them they would benefit from taking this seriously and telling them how sorry they are, instead of defending themselves. The approach should be noncoercive: put forward your own ideas, let clients formulate their own ideas, give them time to think things over and seduce them, as it were, to make sensible proposals about the continuation of treatment (Tennen et al., 1981). It is important that therapists in their descriptions, examples and suggestions are empathic with the ideas and needs of the clients. These clients will then feel that they are understood and will be prepared to accept these words and co-operate (Dhaenens, Schaap, De Mey & Näring, 1989; Van der Velden & Van Dyck, 1977).

The complaining client   These clients, labeled as inhibited, uncertain and submissive (Kiesler, 1983) and masochistic (Leary, 1957), share features of the avoidant and obsessive-compulsive personality disorders of DSM-III-R (APA, 1987). They are rigid, passive and pessimistic. They are ridden by serious and deep-seated conflicts that cannot be solved by other people. They have a need to be assertive but are restrained by chronic doubts, ruminations and inhibitions. They are perfectionists and measure their own faults with high ideals. As a consequence they experience guilt and self-punishment. Their social behaviour is awkward, uncertain and unassertive. In therapy they appeal for help. However, their pessimism and their rigid behaviour pattern is obstructive and may cause discouragement, irritation and impatience among their therapists. This in turn reaffirms their negative self-image. It is important that therapists remain patient, show understanding and interest, and do not raise their expectations too high. The pessimistic client does not feel understood by an optimistic therapist (Leary, 1957). Positive labeling may be more effective (Lange, 1987). These clients also need extrinsic motivation, and therapy should continue in small, concrete steps. Sometimes, an approach is needed in which therapists remain empathic, friendly and understanding, and refrain from instilling hope and pushing the client. Instead, the therapists may become even more passive than the client and only indirectly suggest ways that change may be effected, even though the client is not yet ready.

The dependent client   These clients, often labeled as submissive, trustful (Kiesler, 1983) and dependent–submissive (Leary, 1957), have the features of the dependent personality disorder as distinguished by DSM-III-R (APA, 1987). They are described as experiencing a continuous need for help, affirmation and affection. They usually have few ambitions, few pretensions and little enthusiasm, and tend to overestimate the achievements and capacities of others. In interpersonal contacts they are sensitive and respond strongly to criticism and rejection. They usually find it difficult to formulate their own point of view or to be assertive. They have low self-confidence and have difficulty making decisions or bearing responsibilities. They tend to feel anxious and helpless, and may be motivated in treatment only by being offered a warm and supportive contact. With compliments and positive feedback from the therapist, a dependent client may be encouraged and his or her self-confidence will be strengthened. The therapist may point out the things that have gone well, or the circumstances that caused failures. Assignments may be presented as difficult and therapists may arrange therapy in such a way that these clients get a more active and responsible role. Also, more paradoxical approaches may be taken, for instance, by positively labeling problematic behaviour and by refraining from attacking problematic opinions. Alternatively, the dangers and disadvantages of change may be pointed out.

The foregoing are strategies based on the interpersonal style of the client and must be chosen by the therapist in a relatively early phase of the treatment process to be of benefit to the treatment. The next source for choosing concrete strategies is the quality of the therapeutic relationship, in other words, the way the participants in the treatment process view each other.

The quality of the therapeutic relationship

In an effort to gather strategies to enhance the quality of the therapeutic relationship, Schaap, Hoogduin, Keijsers and Kersten (1989) studied clinical and salesmanship literature. Using handbooks and texts on psychotherapy, social influence, compliance, motivational strategies, resistance, dropout and salesmanship, concrete strategies were gathered. The texts had to comply with the following two criteria: (a) concrete behaviour must be described—an act (e.g., "explaining the therapeutic procedures"), an attitude (e.g., "taking the client's complaints seriously") or an instruction (e.g., "don't be too tolerant when negotiating"); and (b) the behaviour must be characterized by a likelihood of increasing the probability that the client remains in treatment and actively participates in those therapeutic procedures that will lead to improvement.

The selected text units were then rewritten to increase their clarity and had the following form: a definitive therapist behaviour; an eventual explanation; conditions determining the behaviour, including indications and contraindications; examples; and the source reference. From this literature 396 texts were selected, 217 from the clinical and 179 from the salesmanship literature, which are referred to as texts addressing *therapeutic relationship enhancement procedures*.

The next phase involved ordering and classifying the strategies into categories that contained a specific motivating component. The aim was to have a sufficient number of categories in order to be able to present them to therapists and derive the underlying dimensions. This inductive process, based on the literature on common factors described in Chapter 1, yielded 13 categories.

In order to study the underlying structure of these categories, they were presented to 40 therapists who rated them on the basis of similarity. A cluster analysis produced five clusters of activities, which included the original 13 categories. These are outlined below.

Emphasizing expertise
The therapist mobilizes trust of the client in him- or herself   The therapist presents him- or herself as a competent, experienced and reliable person, and increases the client's expectation that his or her problems will be solved. The competent and self-assured therapist behaviour will reassure the client that the therapist will be able to help him or her. A number of factors will determine this reassurance: the client's expectations, information about the therapist and treatment, and the therapist's behaviour.

The therapist promotes trust in the therapeutic procedures   The therapist presents a credible formulation of the presenting problem and a logical explanation of the effective components of the therapeutic procedures.

Giving information   At the onset of treatment, the therapist provides the client with information about the therapy, the procedures and their respective roles.

Enhancing attraction
Unconditional acceptance   The therapist accepts the client, warmly affirms him or her as a person and takes him or her seriously. By conveying this attitude, the therapist promotes a sense of security, which is viewed as a necessary ingredient for therapeutic change.

The therapist is courteous   The therapist treats the client appropriately, in a courteous manner which increases the attraction of the therapeutic relationship. The therapist should be patient, wait for the client to describe a problem, and then summarize and clarify to ensure that it is understood.

The therapist empathizes with the client   The therapist is empathic, interested and enabling, which is expressed in attentive listening as well as in pacing. The therapist should listen attentively and maintain appropriate eye contact; too much eye contact is invasive, too little conveys disinterest.

Establishing a working alliance

The therapist encourages active participation   The therapist encourages the client to adopt an active and participating attitude towards therapy or specific assignments. This active participation increases commitment and compliance, and reduces reactance. The therapist needs to be explicit about the client's participation in treatment (e.g., monitoring and self- observation).

The therapist applies pressure   The therapist maintains the therapeutic tempo by creating agreements or contracts in which the client feels an obligation to participate in the negotiation. The client should be able to present his or her point of view, and any contract should reflect a compromise.

The therapist involves a third party   A positive or participating client attitude is induced by involving a significant other. This category includes all interventions that involve spouses or others in the treatment process, without changing the quality of individual treatment or necessarily initiating marital or family therapy.

Helping with the process of change

The therapist "endorses" the treatment procedure   The therapist tailors the treatment plans to the client's needs and preferences by emphasizing the client's strong points and by matching interventions with client characteristics. The client will feel respected and will expect results from specific therapeutic procedures.

The therapist gives support   The therapist strengthens the client's self-confidence by directing attention to the positive changes that occur and the experiences of learning that are involved. The therapist should be positive, compliment the client, seek positive qualities, try to make the client feel at ease and show encouragement. It is essential to try to increase the client's self-esteem.

The therapist offers help   In contrast to the category above, for which the main emphasis is on increasing the client's self-confidence, the strategies elaborate on the client's problems and complaints, so that the therapist can give advice and help in managing problems.

Utilizing reactance

The therapist utilizes reactance   The therapist copes with the client's unco-operative behaviour by altering the pattern of interaction or using it differently. The therapist might for example respond in such a way that the behaviour pattern can be used to achieve a reduction in complaints. This implies that the therapist accepts the resistance and suggests that the client may not yet be ready for a particular assignment. These strategies can be paradoxical where the therapist deliberately behaves in ways that are different from those which the client expects. The strategies in this category are diverse but they share one important element in that the therapist tries to change the pattern of interaction.

From the above categorization and the concrete strategies gathered in this process, many useful steps have been derived for increasing the motivation of the client to engage in treatment and participate actively. The next two chapters are structured according to the clusters of therapeutic relationship enhancement procedures. However, before turning to these chapters, we will end this chapter by describing some strategies and some examples from case material illustrating how therapists can deal with problems of reactance and non-compliance.

Illustrations of managing problematic situations

Dealing with reactance

Dr Beastly, one of the younger therapists in an outpatient clinic, was known for his low dropout rate. He thought that the reason for this was the fact that he used to be a bouncer in a student nightclub in which he had the capacity to restore order and deal with unruly behaviour without resorting to physical means. In other words, the capacity to influence people in effective ways.

In psychotherapy too, there are people who come for treatment but who do not always behave in ways that therapists may wish. They are dysphoric or aggressive and often do not want to carry out assignments because they already feel overburdened. Therapists who use confrontation will most probably find that their clients stop attending and their dropout rate increase. Other therapists may be more responsive and carefully cope with their client's opinions and ideas, relating to the client acceptance of what he or she brings to the session, and being cautious with directives and advice. Therapists should not wait too long before suggesting an assignment, but it is necessary first to establish a positive therapeutic relationship that would enable tasks to be negotiated. It may also be necessary to refrain from giving assignments if it becomes clear that the client is reluctant to do homework assignments.

This was the case with Mr and Mrs Watts, who came to treatment because they wanted to give up smoking.

Both wanted to quit, according to Mrs Watts, however, it soon became clear that she was the one who wanted to stop. When she was asked what it was worth to her to give up cigarettes, she responded: "at least a thousand pounds because I feel so unhealthy, I have chronic bronchitis and I am a bad example for my children." When her husband was asked the same question, he replied: "Why don't you begin by offering fifty pounds?" Although he was not serious, and it was meant as a joke, it immediately became clear that Mrs Watts was prepared to invest much more in the treatment plan than her husband. It was decided that Mr Watts would continue smoking, under agreed conditions, and that he would be involved in his wife's treatment, for whom success was more important. When his wife indeed succeeded in stopping, his attitude changed and he was prepared to participate fully in treatment as well.

Assessing whether particular advice or an assignment is achievable for a client is probably the most important strategy in preventing relapse or reactance: someone who does not receive a directive cannot oppose it. Some of the methods of assessing client readiness can be carried out with indirect approaches, for example by asking clients how they dealt with the problem in the past. Often some useful strategies are reported, and clients should be complimented for these and encouraged to carry out the strategy in a more systematic way. Clients will then recognize treatment as something for themselves and will be more accepting of it. Such a paradoxical approach (Seltzer, 1986) is not a gimmick or game; depressive clients are not instructed to feel more depressed, rather they are respected for the investment in their fight against depressive symptoms and their morbid thoughts about life, the future and themselves. Respect is the key, and that means that clients will not be forced to do things that they feel are unmanageable at the time; but, simultaneously, positive expectations can be generated.

An important perspective on reactance is the interactional approach (Kiesler, 1982). It is assumed that the client will send the therapist the same rigid and evoking messages that are sent to others. It is the therapist's task to attend to, identify and assess the client's distinctive evoking style as it unfolds within the client-therapist interaction. A major source of this assessment includes the therapist's own emotional and other experiences during these interactions. Here the aim is for both the therapist and client to identify, clarify and establish alternatives to the client's rigid and self-defeating style. The task is to replace these exchanges with more flexible and clear communications that adapt to the changing realities of these specific encounters. The therapist should not respond in the same manner as others, but should give the client the opportunity to experience a different way of interaction. Other suggestions for handling reactance are formulated in the salesmanship literature. McCormack (1984) emphasized that one should recognize one's own limitations and, by doing so, one is more likely to compensate for these, particularly if asked for help rather than insisting on something being done. The other person will then feel respected and will be more likely to alter their interaction style.

Our basic message is that the presentation of therapeutic techniques is as important as the techniques themselves. There is an important aspect of interventions that is relevant to this discussion. Interventions vary on three bipolar dimensions; they can be literal or metaphorical, direct or indirect, and congruent or paradoxical. We will focus primarily on this latter distinction.

Usually psychotherapeutic interventions are literal; if we want a client to carry out a particular assignment, we explain it, negotiate around it and formulate how it should be conducted. In the case of Mr Jones described earlier, the behavioural treatment of obsessive-compulsive symptoms required him to monitor the extent to which the symptoms occurred. The rationale was explained and he was then requested to monitor his symptoms. The therapist, however, could have used a different approach: the treatment rationale could have been explained and then, instead of asking him to monitor his behaviour, the therapist could have used the "client metaphor", i.e., he could have described another client, similar to Mr Jones, who had developed his own way of keeping track of his symptoms. What one essentially does in such a situation is create an atmosphere that increases the likelihood of the client responding appropriately.

Interventions also differ in the way they are supposed to achieve their aim. In assertiveness training, we can ask a client to show particular assertive responses, but we could also manipulate certain environmental factors, which could increase the likelihood of these responses. In modelling a situation presented by one of the participants in group assertiveness training, another member could be "seduced" to play the role of a talkative bar-keeper, a role he or she would never actually play in real life.

Interventions also vary on a congruence–paradox dimension. It is congruent to tell Mr Jones that we will try to reduce his obsessive-compulsive behaviour by making it increasingly difficult for him to exhibit it. It is paradoxical to tell him to exhibit more obsessive-compulsive behaviour or to resist the therapist's attempts to get him to monitor his behaviour, for instance, by using the rationale that he has to become more independent.

Reactance can be used therapeutically, and therapists should be aware that it *can* be used towards positive ends. For this reason, it should be accepted. Failing to do so implies to the client that it is something negative and to be avoided. The therapist should make it clear to clients that, when they try out new behaviours, this does not necessarily imply that they should give up their old ways. The therapist may even encourage a client to exhibit old problematic patterns of behaviour and at the same time, present new and more effective ones. It may also be useful to present an assignment not as something easily mastered, but as a challenge. The therapist may even suggest that the client is not ready for a particular assignment, thereby stimulating him or her to demonstrate that he or she has been underestimated.

The therapist may go further and tell the client the assignment is difficult, perhaps even too difficult and that he/she may need some time to think about it. This will emphasize to the client that therapeutic assignments are a challenge and will thus increase client's self-confidence when they do experience a sign of mastery. The therapist may also label the symptoms as an ordeal, thereby making it more difficult for the client to continue with the symptomatic behaviour. It is advisable for the therapist to have a good understanding and formulation of the processes involved in the client's presentation and possibly even mention that the current difficulties may serve to improve the situation. This will place clients in a dilemma in that they will have to consider the functional nature of the symptom, which may well render it less attractive.

A number of clients are likely to resist suggestions when placed in a social influence situation such as psychotherapy. Here the therapist may try to increase reactance by being directive, persuasive, emphasizing their status as an expert and minimizing the client's freedom of choice, while at the same time maintaining an optimal therapeutic relationship. The therapist may also utilize the reactance by labeling it in an opposite way; for example, with a rigid and controlling client, the therapist may say the assignment fits in well with the client's spontaneous and flexible way of responding.

A paradoxical intervention can take the form of prescribing the symptomatic behaviour, something that clients find confusing and difficult to accept. The confusion need not necessarily be seen negatively, because it requires the client to consider ways of resolving the dilemma, which often then induces change. Clients who are particularly suspicious of therapy, who wish to engage in a power struggle with the therapist or who think they know better, are likely to show reactance. The therapist should not insist that they take up the option of therapy, but rather should agree with them by indicating a degree of pessimism and the small likelihood of a positive outcome. The therapist should nevertheless emphasize the serious nature of the symptoms and remain modest about his or her own abilities. Criticism about the therapist and other members of the helping profession can then be labeled positively as an indication of a critical attitude and a reluctance to follow suggestions immediately, which could be labeled as a sign of independence.

This discussion on dealing with client reactance is essentially based on ideas from the literature on paradox. On the one hand, clients are presented with a counter-paradox, but on the other hand it is the reluctant or defensive client who presents with the original paradox: "help me, but I do not want to change". By introducing a counter-paradox, the client chooses whether to maintain their position or to opt for a different one by using therapy to overcome that element of the paradox described as "but I do not want to change". To illustrate this approach, some examples are presented below.

Case illustrations

The incompetent therapist

Mr T., a male client diagnosed as having a panic disorder with agoraphobia does not respond to such congruent therapeutic interventions as relaxation exercises, hyperventilation provocation, cue-conditioning and exposure. Instead, there is an aggravation of the symptomatology. Since an authority conflict characterized the relationship between Mr T. and his therapist, the therapist decides to build upon this issue and give Mr T. a greater sense of power in their relationship. The therapist does this by emphasizing her own mistakes to Mr T. She apologizes to him for her obviously ineffective approach and her poor choice of treatment technique. Within 15 minutes of such talk, Mr T. responds, "You are not important to me anyway, I don't need you, I have already improved considerably." Their sessions continue in this fashion and after three sessions of such an innovative approach, there is a significant diminishing of the complaints. He ends his therapy, telling the therapist that he would be alright as long as she stayed clear from him.

Holidays

Mr J. presents himself as lonesome and depressed. He demonstrates very little initiative in trying to come to grips with and improving his quality of life. In order to overcome his apathy, his therapist feels that Mr J. should go on a holiday. In order to mobilize Mr J. he advises him in a very indirect way, "Obviously a holiday would be the best thing for you right now, it would allow you the time to leave your problems behind you for a while and get a fresh perspective on things. But I really don't think at this moment in your condition that it is possible for you to get away, so don't even consider it right now. It would be too much for you I feel. Perhaps in a couple of days you will be ready to consider it but we must really wait and see." Mr J. responds immediately with great enthusiasm to the idea of going on a holiday; he demonstrates his interest by beginning to discuss several issues related to planning a holiday. In a later stage of the therapy sessions, again, Mr J. is advised to remain calm and realistic about his holiday plans given his condition. Immediately, Mr J. becomes more energetic and expressive and his plans to go on a holiday become more concrete.

The good listener

Mr S. presents himself in an extremely dull way. He is, amongst other things, unable to conduct an interesting discussion. His therapist emphasizes that for a good conversation two parties are needed, a speaker and a listener. Instead of the therapist trying to change Mr S.'s dull manner and presentation, she focuses on his listening skills. She tells him, "It is not necessary that you make an interesting conversation; some people are simply good listeners." She advises him to begin monitoring his listening behaviour: active listening, good eye contact, and paraphrasing. The result of having him focus on his listening skills was an immediate decrease in his worrying about being a good speaker, and thus a more lively involvement characterized Mr S. when interacting with others.

The neurological disease
Ms R. has been diagnosed with a conversion paralysis of her legs and panic disorder. She has made it clear to her husband that she does not want to do anything to help with the upkeep of the household. She also does not want to have sex with him any more. Her manner in presenting these wishes to her husband are quite passive–aggressive as she typically phrases her wishes as: "I would like to, but my illness makes it impossible." She has a very critical attitude towards the world, her husband and the therapist included. For the treatment, the therapist feels that it is important to keep Ms R. in the patient role for the time being, with the following rationale: "Ms R., you have an uncommon neurological disease. You will have to spare yourself: do not strain yourself in the household, you should refrain from any sexual contact, you need good physiotherapy to further loosen your legs and, very importantly, you will need an "overdose" of rest during the day." This intervention leads to a situation where the panic disappears completely and Ms R. is able to walk for some hundred metres. The foundation of further treatment is thus laid.

A candle burning at both ends
Mr M., a client diagnosed with burnout, tends to dominate the exchange between himself and his therapist. The therapist feels he is thus unable to gather the necessary information he would like for the treatment plan. To change this interaction, the therapist starts off with complimentary and empathic remarks to Mr M.: "You have suffered a lot. You have survived extremely well the hideous bosses you have had." The therapist then asks a closed question. When Mr M. continues his lamentation, the therapist breaks in and gives a short summary and says to Mr M. "You have suffered so much, you are like a candle burning at both ends, it would be a shame if you forgot to tell me some of your experiences in this short time we have together, could you write everything down and send it to me?" With this instruction, the therapist regained control of the sessions.

Life is war
Mr V., is a client diagnosed with panic attacks and agoraphobia and has completed a hyperventilation programme for his symptoms. He still fears losing control: "I am afraid of fainting. I am afraid that when I am talking with an acquaintance I will not be able to find the right words for what I want to say." The therapeutic programme results in a situation where he is able to manage his symptoms and his life. However, he still considers life threatening: he conducts a continuous war against other people. The therapist agrees with Mr V.'s view of a hostile world, and provides personal examples of how people have wounded him as well, and that bureaucracy is a particularly easy target for such attacks. He advises Mr V., "Do not let down your guard at any time, at the same time don't let those turkeys get you down. Try and be nice to them and that way you will get on top of them. Watch other people and see how they get things done. Observe and use the strategies that you see are effective." This results in an improvement in the therapeutic relationship and a phase where Mr

V. is able to work with the therapist on his perception of others around him.

Life is shit
Ms A., complains of extreme headaches and pain in her arm and knee. Sometimes she has crying spells and aggressive outbursts during which she breaks everything in her room to smithereens. She also complains of considerable marital problems. She uses her therapy hour to complain about the lack of affection she received in her youth and her attempts to gain affection from others in her adult life. Her passive attitude seduces the therapist and her husband to suggest ways to arrive at some happiness in her life. Again and again she succeeds in proving that this advice is worthless. Then, the therapist changes his behaviour, explicitly listens to her complaints, shows respect for her complaints and her endurance. He compliments her about her amazing stamina to endure such hardship, and suggests to her that she will not be able to follow the programme that he had in mind for her. He says to her, "It is a pity that you can not follow the programme that I had planned for you, it is certainly a very effective treatment plan, particularly with strong people who are able to keep things up. Your suffering is yet too severe, I'm afraid." The patient reacts by then slowly changing her need to be a martyr.

"Therapeutic massage"
During the intake session, a solicitor, Mr B., who has been diagnosed with depression and panic attacks, elaborates on how perfect he is in contrast with all the people surrounding him. He says to his therapist, "My superiors never listen to my good ideas, they are so blind, and my clients, they don't listen to me either they are obstinate and real nincompoops." He is quite capable of solving his hyperventilation problem by telling himself: "Okay, if my days are counted, then I should die." When the therapist summarizes to Mr B., his problems, he gives an inaccurate summary. Mr B. is always in turn successful in finding little points that the therapist overlooked. The therapist then decides to change his strategy. When the patient tells him that he can manage and control his hyperventilation attack within 20 minutes, the therapist immediately expresses his surprise and tells the client that most patients can't, and that he admires the inventiveness of the client. When the client again tells the therapist that his boss does not listen to him, the therapist tells him empathically that that is often the case with those "fallen up" people—small bosses who want to play God in their little enterprises. The therapist then suggests to the patient that, although he mastered his complaints to a large extent, there might be some additional points where he could use some advice. At the same time he suggests that some patients are opinionated, just like the patient's clients. Therapy can only be successful if patients co-operate and think with the therapist critically about the best way to change. Then the therapist mentions a number of practical suggestions and continues asking the patient what he considers a sensible thing to do. The therapist continues to tell the patient that he really considers him not as a patient but rather as a colleague, and suggests that a small number of instructive sessions would probably not hurt. During the following sessions, conducted in roughly the same way, the therapist has no further problems with this patient.

In the following two chapters we will focus more extensively on strategies to engage the client in therapy and to maintain a collaborative set. These strategies are derived mainly from the study on therapeutic relationship enhancement procedures, described earlier.

4 Engaging the client

Introduction

Mr Smith, a 55-year-old instrument maker, was referred to an outpatient clinic for panic attacks, depression and psychosomatic stomach complaints. Four years earlier, he had undergone heart surgery. Mr Smith is a small man who reported in detail a series of traumatic events which he experienced and which he felt were caused by other people. He was quite hostile, sarcastic and became emotional when talking about a period, 10 years earlier, when his wife "had a nervous breakdown". At about this time, a friend not only seduced his wife but also managed to "terrorize" his family and threaten him. This led him to experience serious financial hardship and family problems. He agreed that, perhaps as a result of this, he is difficult to get along with. He further acknowledged having many interpersonal problems.

A number of psychological tests were used during the assessment. His scores on the psychological tests indicated that he was rather dogmatic and had a distrustful and paranoid attitude. The Symptom Checklist (SCL-90; Arrindel & Ettema, 1986; Deragotis, 1977)) showed elevated scores on almost all scales when compared to the norm group of psychiatric patients. The profile indicated a sense of vulnerability and personal inadequacy when with others.

It was explained to Mr Smith that he would have to wait 2 months before starting therapy. The therapist suggested that in the meantime, he could start treatment on his own using a self-control procedure, which is only suggested to strong and competent clients. With his curiousity aroused, he wanted more information about the treatment. He was told that it was a very difficult approach, and would involve again coping with the earlier traumatic events at the time of his wife's problems, by writing a continuous letter. The therapist explained that this procedure would require him to go to his study at a particular time of the day and look at photographs and other memories of that difficult period of his life. When his emotions were aroused, he was to write down everything that came to his mind. After a fixed time period, half an hour was suggested, his wife was to come upstairs, stop him from writing and together they should have a drink. The therapist explained that it was important to find something to do that would be incompatible with worrying and would interrupt his continuous letter. It was agreed that he and his wife would play cards as this would be a good distraction for him. Two weeks later, Mr Smith called the therapist to say that he had started the self-control procedure and to ask whether he was doing it correctly. The therapist emphasized that he should not be concerned about his language or style but ensure that he wrote whatever came to his mind. The therapist again emphasized again that the treatment was tough, but that he was certain Mr Smith could do it.

When the therapy sessions started 2 months later, Mr Smith confidently reported to the therapist that he had overcome his problem for the most part, but that he needed still some help, particularly with his marital problems.

In the previous chapter, we presented evidence for and described the problem of dropout, particularly following the intake interview. Since this is common, it is important that deliberate attempts are made to ensure that the clients return for a second appointment, particularly if treatment has to be delayed. The case described above illustrates how the intake interview can be used in engaging a client by showing the therapist's expertise and ideas, thereby creating a positive therapeutic atmosphere. The therapist should not be sidetracked by the seriousness of the complaints nor should they be dismissed; instead, the therapist should increase his/her attractiveness by using humour, by empathic listening, by being courteous and by trying to share the client's general perceptions.

In this chapter we will describe some therapeutic relationship enhancement procedures that can be of use to engage clients in the therapeutic process. The concrete procedures centre around the concepts of the therapist's expertise and the appeal of attraction of the therapeutic relationship.

Expertise

The therapist's expertise is based on the socially sanctioned role of healer. In creating the therapist's expert position, we focus on the concrete behaviours that play a role in developing this perception. By way of introduction, we will summarize some results essentially from studies on nonverbal communication and impression management, and will go on to discuss the dimensions of the therapist's expert status.

Nonverbal cues of impression management, persuasion and dominance

Cappella and Street (1985) described the nonverbal behaviour that is used when people try to impress one another. In an initial encounter such as an intake interview, persons interacting often show stereotypical desirable behaviour. A variety of nonverbal cues are associated with success in creating a favourable impression such as rapid and fluent speech, many utterances with relatively few pauses, short latency times, a standard accent, speech that is not too loud or too soft, lexical diversity and good eye contact (Street & Hopper, 1982). Patterson (1982) and Knapp (1978) suggest that the psychotherapist's perceived expertise is enhanced by an increase in looking at the client, leaning forward, directing gestures towards the client, showing facial expressiveness, nodding and using interpretative utterances.

Another important group of relevant nonverbal cues are persuasion or compliance enhancing tactics. Nonverbal styles of communication become more frequent when attempting to be persuasive: looking at another, nodding, facial expressiveness, loudness and rate of speech all tend to increase. Attitude changes are usually observed as a result of persuasion when speech rate increases, language use is intense, different lexical choices are observed, accents are matched between the respondents and where verbal and nonverbal behaviour is consistent (Apple, Streeter & Kraus, 1979; Bradac, Brower & Courtright, 1979; Dabbs, 1969; Giles & Powesland, 1975).

A further important dimension in social interaction and of relevance to expertise is dominance. Patterson (1982) reviewed the literature on nonverbal cues and suggested that in stable relationships, the following cues are associated with the more powerful person: the actor looks more at the partner when he/she is speaking than vice versa; the actor looks less at the partner when listening; the actor touches the other person more, is less facially expressive and is more relaxed. If the power relations are being negotiated, then those who are perceived as more powerful will show more interruptions, more and faster speech, more touch and more variation in lexical style (Major & Haslin, 1982; Rogers & Jones, 1975; Scherer, 1979; Shaw, 1981).

Promoting trust in the person of the therapist

Mrs Langley, a 49-year-old deaf divorcee living on a government allowance, was referred to an outpatient clinic for panic attacks and depression. She had had several rows with the secretary of the outpatient clinic prior to her intake session. She had on several occasions changed the appointment of her initial assessment and requested that she should be seen at a time that was convenient to her. When the secretary understandably and carefully explained the problem of arranging appointments, she started complaining about how everybody, particularly doctors, made her life so miserable; eventually, however, an appropriate time was agreed upon.

During the intake session, Mrs Langley immediately started to complain about all the physicians who had not taken her seriously. The assessor agreed with her noting the disinterest and incompetence of some of the medical profession, particularly those specializing in her particular problems. He pointed out the success of the outpatient clinic with patients presenting with panic attacks like hers, without being overly optimistic. She then described at length her many difficulties, which included deafness, social isolation, her parents forcing her to marry a man she did not love and the consequent divorce, having to raise her only daughter alone and the death of a friendly neighbour. It was obvious that Mrs Langley was very unhappy yet instead of reflecting this, the therapist suggested that she "was a very strong and resilient woman." When she asked abruptly how this could be, the therapist pointed out that someone who had survived so much, must be strong and resourceful. She was surprised and obviously taken off guard by the comment. She told the therapist that she was often self-dismissive and told herself that she was "an old bat and a good for nothing." The therapist suggested that she should change her self-talk and instead tell herself that she was a strong person. After he found out that she was a religious person, he told her to repeat the sentence from the bible "a strong woman who shall find her". The therapist then suggested that she also had a great sense of humour; she again asked how this could be, to which the therapist told her that he could tell because of the glistening in her eyes. At that point she told the therapist, mischievously, that her eyes could glisten even more.

The therapist then withdrew and let Mrs Langley formulate the most appropriate treatment for her problems. She started to explain how she needed coaching in trying to relax so she could perceive the world differently. The therapist intervened and explained she should remain distrustful telling her, "You cannot trust other people, you have to solve your problems on your own; stay aloof and only start to trust other people when they have provided you with the evidence that you can do so." He then used a "client metaphor" and described ways that other patients had been helped by coping with their anxiety and panic attacks and regaining control over their lives.

At the end of the intake session, Mrs Langley was told that there would be a 2 month wait before treatment could start. He then formulated some interventions that would lead to increased relaxation and enhance her capacity to cope with anxiety and panic. An important component of her self-control treatment programme consisted of keeping a daily activity diary that would be used when treatment commenced. At the same time she agreed to use self-statements that implied that she was a strong woman, and the conditions that reinforced her maintaining her side of the bargain were then discussed.

Frank (1982) emphasized the importance of the therapist's reputation, expertise and prestige as a way of presenting self-confidence, which creates hope and positive expectations. Frank also mentioned the actual setting and suggested having books and displaying certificates to emphasize status. This situation then promotes an atmosphere of security and positive expectations, conveying to clients that they will be taken seriously, will be listened to and that the therapy is trustworthy and safe. The therapist's expertise can also be enhanced by outlining the number of patients who have had the treatment. And some accounts of therapeutic successes.

Expertise will also be increased by predicting associated symptoms. If a client with panic attacks based on hyperventilation, describes symptoms of breathlessness and choking, it may be worthwhile to describe other symptoms such as dizziness, palpitations, a dry throat, and cold hands and feet. With a depressive client, the therapist might predict the loss of appetite and the resulting weight loss, or feelings of guilt and remorse. Similarly, if a client describes perfectionism, to predict that he/she will not start something if he/she knows it cannot be done perfectly, will enhance the perception of the therapist's expertise.

Some procedures can be inferred from the social psychological literature on influencing processes (McGuire, 1985; Wrightsman & Deaux, 1981). The therapist may wish to warn the clients about other people's attempts to influence them, and encourage the clients to be more decisive. It is also important that the message is clear and is formulated several times with slightly different emphases. It is useful to use analogy and comparisons that focus attention and create favourable expectancies. A number of concrete strategies have been formulated in the salesmanship literature (e.g., Borgeest, 1958; McCormack, 1984). Competence can be conveyed by being self-assured, taking the initiative while at the same time maintaining some distance.

Enhancing trust in the therapeutic procedures

Mrs Ramsey, a 35-year-old married midwife, was referred to an outpatient clinic for panic attacks. Her first attack had occurred 6 months earlier while she was driving her car. She had suddenly panicked, and had had to stop the car and wait for about an hour before she was able to continue, and only then could she proceed with extreme anxiety. She subsequently developed a fear of travelling by car on her own. She was, however, quite an independent person and the avoidance was the primary reason for her referral to the clinic. She maintained that the attacks were inconsistent with her self-image as a competent, independent woman. During the intake session she explained that at the time of her panic attack, she was having problems at work which she was unable to ignore. At the same time her father, with whom she was very close, had become ill and died a few months later. Her scores on the psychological tests did not indicate other serious difficulties, but she did have relatively high scores on anxiety and agoraphobia.

It was explained to Mrs Ramsey that her panic attacks were hyperventilation attacks caused by a loss of carbon dioxide. It was also suggested to her that she was under a great deal of stress at the time of her first attack and that she reacted to the stress by hyperventilating. She spontaneously offered the idea that she would have to get used to telling herself that a hyperventilation attack was imminent, instead of thinking that something awful was about to happen. The hyperventilation provocation test was explained to her and she was told that she would be requested to hyperventilate in the therapist's office in order to be taught how to stop the attack. She would then be asked to practice the provocation at home with her husband. The final step of treatment would involve an exposure procedure of driving her car alone again. Following this explanation, Mrs Ramsey agreed with the therapist and indicated that she had already anticipated the nature of the treatment.

It is important that the therapist offers credible explanations for the presenting symptoms and gives a logical explanation of the effective components of the treatment. The rationale for the symptoms and related problems will reduce anxiety and helplessness. Some therapists also offer the client a diagnosis, for example, explaining to an obsessive-compulsive patient that he/she is suffering from an anxiety disorder and that the compulsion is a way of dealing with and neutralizing fear.

Obviously, the credible rationale is somewhat problematic in cases where client and therapist differ with regard to the cause of the problem, as for instance in the case of a somatic disorder. Nevertheless, there as well, the therapist should try and get close to the client's conceptualization. This can be expressed in statements like: "There might have been or there is a somatic basis for your complaint. However, since the medical specialist can't help you, we will focus on the stress that increases your suffering."

Giving information

Mr Peterson and his wife were referred to the clinic because of their marital problems. At the core of these problems was his bipolar disorder. Over the previous 5 years, he had experienced three manic episodes during which he would become impulsive, dominating and even violent. He had also recently bought a house, which the family could not really afford. These periods, which lasted for a couple of months, alternated with periods when he isolated himself and became very depressed. Careful questioning about what had happened, revealed the following: Mr Peterson held a very responsible job at an executive level for a multinational company, until 5 years previously when he was unexpectedly made redundant. A difficult period followed, involving solicitors; however, in the end, he left the company on medical grounds and obtained a disability allowance from the government. It was at this point that he had his first period of depression and received some therapeutic help. Soon after beginning treatment, he had another manic period and was given lithium as the preferred treatment for bipolar disorders. However, the psychiatrist did not explain that he would possibly have to take lithium for the rest of his life. His wife was not invited to attend any sessions and was not even told what to expect. After some time Mr Peterson stopped the lithium, precipitating a second manic episode. Again it was prescribed and, again, he stopped taking it. Finally, the couple were referred for marital therapy on the wife's initiative. His wife insisted on him complying with the lithium regime. An appointment was made for the couple to see the psychiatrist from the lithium clinic, who explained the details of bipolar disorder to them, explaining that it was clear that Mr Peterson would have to take the lithium for the foreseeable future. The marital therapy, which began after correct lithium levels had been established, indeed had a good outcome.

It is important that the therapist carefully describes the treatment and the therapeutic procedures and gives information about the cause of the disorder and related problems. It is also advisable to illustrate the different steps of the treatment using examples from case material, thereby demonstrating how symptoms can be reduced. In the treatment of panic attacks with agoraphobia, it can be explained to the client how the attacks are triggered. This explanation may suggest a number of necessary treatment steps to reduce the levels of arousal.

The pace of providing information is crucial because offering too much or too threatening material before clients are able to accept it could make it difficult for them to return. When clients do not define their difficulties, such as marital problems, and are hesitant to admit relationship distress, doing so too soon can have disadvantages.

Mr and Mrs Robinson were referred to a community mental health centre following his panic attacks. When they first came to the office, the assessor told them that Mr Robinson's problems reflected marital problems and that marital therapy was the preferred treatment. Mr Robinson then got up, said that their car was illegally parked, and never returned.

Such a case may be encountered if a strict mono-treatment approach is taken. Even if this assessor was right in attributing the marital relationship of the Robinsons as the cause or determinant of the panic attacks, it surely did not make Mr Robinson feel understood.

Perhaps, the best known format for providing information can be found in the psychosocial treatment of schizophrenia. In psychoeducative programmes, relatives of schizophrenic patients are given detailed information about the incidence, the possible causes and the available treatment (e.g., Falloon, Boyd & McGill, 1984). Such information often includes descriptions of ways a family can reduce stress and cope with difficult and unpredictable behaviour of the patient. The provision of information, involving others in the treatment of a family member, increases their coping responses and reduces the secrecy and myths that often exist in psychological and psychiatric treatments.

Attractiveness: interventions based on the relationship inventory

In the early 1950s, Carl Rogers formulated his ideas about accurate empathy, non-possessive warmth and genuineness being necessary and sufficient conditions for psychotherapeutic change. Cappella and Street (1985) have described the behavioural cues that increase the social attractiveness within psychotherapeutic encounters. It can be assumed that the quality of the therapeutic relationship is influenced positively to the extent that the therapist displays behaviours linked to showing expertise. Patterson (1982) and Knapp (1978) reported that trust and warmth are increased by facial expressiveness, gestures directed towards the patient, looking at the patient, changes in posture, open hand movements and relatively little talking.

Since Rogers' pioneering work, much research has been conducted by his students. It is possible to conclude that the Rogerian conditions seem to be necessary in effecting therapeutic change, but that their impact and generalizability are not as great as was once thought. There is, however, no evidence to assume that the conditions are sufficient for therapeutic change irrespective of the treatment approach. Certainly, the Rogerian conditions are necessary and particularly so during the beginning phase of treatment, but they are not sufficient as treatment factors alone. Because of their importance, we will consider some strategies that enhance attractiveness based on these Rogerian conditions.

The fundamental idea behind therapeutic relationship enhancement procedures is that the clients themselves provide the information necessary to determine which procedures are most useful. One of the instruments that provides this information (and is further described in Chapter 6) is the Relationship Inventory (RI; Barrett-Lennard, 1962). On the basis of negative scores on the RI, clients indicate what procedures would lead to a more positive perception of the therapeutic relationship. Therapists can then be approached and asked to indicate the extent to which particular procedures would lead to a more positive therapeutic relationship as perceived by clients. Schaap and Hoogduin (1988) reviewed the literature on therapeutic relationship enhancement procedures and then tried to match the RI questions with a number of intuitively relevant procedures. These were then presented to 20 therapists, requesting that they indicate which of the procedures would lead to more positive scores. Below we present a list of items from the RI and, for each, the specific relationship enhancement procedures that the respondents suggested would be effective in achieving a more positive client score on that particular aspect of the relationship:

The therapist does not appreciate what goes on inside of me:
- accurately formulate and convey the feelings and responses of clients,
- try to use the clients' words, expressions and images,
- tell clients that you can imagine everything that they have suffered,
- tell clients that you respect their perseverance,
- adapt your speech rate to that of the client.

I make the therapist nervous:
- remain calm and relaxed,
- do not fidget or play with objects,
- be friendly and good humoured,
- smile from time to time,
- let the clients finish their stories,
- invite clients to talk about themselves by asking, for example, how they solved problems in the past,
- give compliments and express your appreciation.

The therapist does not like to see me:
- give compliments and express your appreciation,
- tell clients that they can be helped by talking about problems and that you would like to help them in this process,
- show your interest and commitment, for example, by making relevant reading material available,

- encourage clients to talk about themselves and acknowledge what they say,
- go into the subject that clients talk about, even if it is not directly related to therapy.

The therapist considers me a bore and of little interest:
- attend to your nonverbal behaviour, in particular eye contact,
- compliment your client and express your appreciation,
- go into the material your client brings, even it has little to do with therapy,
- never reject the clients' ideas,
- ask extensively about their complaints,
- ask about their positive qualities,
- surprise clients by your detailed knowledge of their background, e.g., showing that the case notes have been carefully read.

Engaging clients is most probably the key to most positive therapeutic outcomes. If successfully achieved, compliance will be enhanced, the risk of dropout will be reduced and the client will co-operate to the extent that he or she still has positive expectations. There are methods that can be utilized to promote engagement and they should be seen as an essential part of therapeutic relationships. We conclude this chapter with a verbatim intake session, illustrating some of the relationship enhancement procedures described earlier.

A verbatim illustration of motivating strategies

The client is a 40-year-old married woman presenting an obsessive-compulsive disorder. She and her husband were invited for the following assessment session. The therapist begins by explaining that the session will be videotaped and then continues explaining what the patient and her husband can expect. He also requests their co-operation in participating in an empirical investigation, and uses a structured interview schedule.

Initially, the therapist tries to get information to make the right assessment of the complaint. The motivating strategy of this vignette is the therapist repeating or recapping what the client is saying, but doing so in his own words, showing his expertise and generating trust.

Th. Could you please tell me what your main complaint is?
C. I have, when I clean something, it is mainly when I clean something, you see, this wallet has to go into my purse, the purse is closed and then I will open it many times, and then I watch my wallet, okay it is well inside, purse closed, purse open, yes, the wallet is inside, purse closed, and that continues several times.
Th. How many times is "several times"?
C. Some days it can be 28 times.
Th. And in half an hour?

C.   If I am lucky, three times

H.   But usually it is bad luck.

Th. The question is why do you do that? What thoughts force you to do so?

C.   Because I think that it is not right. I put it in, zip up, open the purse to see if it is inside and well, yes it is, yes, but then another look to make sure.

Th. If it is not right, then what?

C.   Then there is nothing the matter, is there?!

Th. Yes, but I am asking you?

C.   Well, I don't know.

Th. But then you have this thought, it emerges: it is not right, then a kind of tension emerges, a kind of compulsive feeling . . . you experience a kind of insecurity: is it alright? Then you check it again or really repeat it, or do you only check? Do you only look into your purse or do you have to put the wallet in it again?

C.   No, I will show you. I put the wallet in, close the purse, open it and check, close it again, open it again, close it, and so on. So, I keep the wallet in the purse.

Th. Exactly, you do not have to repeat the act. The important thing is the checking. And sometimes you have to repeat certain things but that is only because otherwise it is impossible to check. Do you understand? You open your purse and close it each time, that is only a repetition to see if it still is inside. Suppose you decided that it would be sufficient to put it on the table. Then you could be satisfied with looking at it, to see if it is still there. Then you would not have to go towards it, take it and put it back. So there is an insecurity: you try to solve that by saying to yourself: now it is right!

C.   Yes.

The therapist is trying to involve the husband in the client's problems thereby increasing pressure. He is also predicting what is happening, indicating his expertise which will hopefully increase trust.

Th. Do you sometimes ask your husband for help?

H.   Often if things have to be put away in cupboards or so, then I walk with her to the cupboard.

Th. Is she then satisfied with doing it once?

H.   No! Then I open the cupboard and close it again and then she says: "Open it again!" So I open it again.

Th. So, it is a kind of reassurance? It doesn't really help, and it probably helped more in the beginning than it does now?

C.   Yes.

In addition the fact that the following is an important distinction in the sense that the client shows a compulsion or a cognitive activity, the therapist is demonstrating his expertise and knowledge of the complaint.

Th. Exactly! . . . Is it also the case that you repeat an act in thought? For instance, you have put something in your purse and you then leave. And then in your thoughts you try to imagine how it was and if it was right. You put your iron away and, for instance, if you are in your car, you check your thoughts: "Have I put it there, in such a way, yes." Is this how it is?

By exaggerating the co-operation and reassurance provided by the husband, the therapist is assessing the client's motivation to solve her problems and investigates the secondary gain. The utterance is delivered in a pleasant, even humorous way, and will certainly increase the attractiveness of the therapist.

C. Yes, I can, as my husband says, continue nagging. Yes, it is nagging, really.
Th. You mean, to go back and check?
C. Oh yes, that is what I would really like to do. My husband does an awful lot for me, but not that, yet.
Th. Not yet? Do you mean that one of these days he will have to do so?
C. Oh no, hope not.

Here the therapist is being empathic, as well as directive. He is implying that the client has been suffering and is still doing so, but that a solution for her problems is possible.

H. When I return from work and I lock the car door and a couple of minutes later she will check if the door is really locked. And at night, I have to do it again.
Th. So you get really involved? And you are also sometimes used to give reassurance, to tell your wife, that everything is alright?
H. Yes.
Th. How long have you had these complaints?
C. In June, 21 years.
Th. Then it is time we did something about it.

This is an important point in this conversation. The therapist is again assessing the client's motivation for following a treatment programme, particularly the intensity of her distress.

Th. Okay, let's summarize what we have so far. You have a thought that catches you: "Something is not right, I have not done something the right way."
C. Yes.
Th. Then you check and if that is impossible, for instance because you are in the car, then you check everything in your mind. You also get your husband involved. Any other person besides your husband?

C. My sister came during the summer to pick me up and the children. They were on holiday and she knows what is the matter with me. I took care that everything was prepared and that everything had been checked. I then called her inside and walked with her through the whole house from top till bottom. Windows closed, gas turned off. She really just accompanied me to show me that everything is alright. The front door closed. And also my mother. But otherwise no one. They are the only ones.

Th. You do have children?

C. Yes, twins, eight years old.

Th. Any problems with the children?

C. No, everything is fine, and financially we are well off.

Th. So, no catastrophes?

C. No, I wish I could buy it off. Not that I have the capital to do so.

Th. How much do you offer? Not seriously of course. I will return to this later because I am going to ask you how much it is worth to you. Not that we are going to bill you, you do not have to be afraid of that, but to get an indication how bad things are.

Here again the client is expressing her high positive expectations. The therapist indicates that the therapy programme is tailored to her needs thereby endorsing the treatment procedure.

H. During the last weeks things have gotten worse.

Th. Worse?

C. I feel as if I am going to a party when I come here.

H. At least you have the idea that something can be done about it.

Th. That is so. The next appointments are already fixed. So you can start with the therapy programme right away.

The therapist is empathic, indicating that he understands that the couple must experience some tension in their marriage as a result of the wife's compulsion. Again he does so in a humorous way, increasing his attractiveness and resulting in disclosure.

Th. How is your relationship? The complaints must put a strain on your marriage. How are the two of you getting along?

H. No problem, is there?

C. No.

Th. You look at each other in a certain way?!

Here the therapist is empathic, on the one hand recognizing the severity of the complaints, while also showing the client the important things that make her life worthwhile.

C: Well, I am not the most sociable person at home, I know that. I mean I can stand with red eyes at the door, or I cannot stand much. Also towards the children. And then I say: "Well, it is no problem for you." And then you might get some problems. He is sometimes fed up with it. He also has his job.

H. Like on Monday, I came home at 5.15 pm and we had been away for a couple of days, so we had to check a number of things. We only finished at 11.30 pm, just before midnight.

C. Yes, we had not had time to sit down.

Th. What do you think about all this checking?

C. Disgusting!

Th. Do you think it is all nonsense?

C. Yes, total nonsense.

Th. That makes it doubly bad, because if it has some sense . . . But now you think: "What am I doing?"

C. Yes, awful. I also think about all these lost years. They can never be repeated.

Th. What you have had you have had. But there were also nice things as well, weren't there?

C. Sure, two healthy kids, a lovely husband, nice parents. I have enough, I really have everything I want. I don't have any other problems.

This is important. The therapist shows his attractiveness and his expertise. He is indicating that the symptoms give the client a kind of purpose in life, even if they are experienced negatively. It is also implied, more explicitly elsewhere that there are many areas in her life that are symptom-free.

Th. But you really don't have any time for other problems.

C. No, that is true.

Again the therapist is assessing the client's motivation to participate in the treatment programme. He is also responding with humour to her, referring to a woman's magazine, showing his attraction as a person and as a professional.

Th. How did your problems start?

H. At one particular minute, wasn't it?

C. One second!

Th. What happened exactly?

C. That was during secondary school. I was studying and our neighbour came in and said: "Mary [that is a friend of mine] has passed her exams and it was a beautiful party, with flowers, and so on." And I thought: "Oh yeah." I had to do my exam the next day. I stood up and wanted to study outside, because it was summer. I walked passed the kitchen table, and I thought I had to touch it because I had to pass that exam. That was what I really wanted. And that is how it came about. It just shot in.

Th. Yes I understand . . .

Th. You said that you did not come here because your GP or husband said so, but because you wanted to . . . How did you say?

C. I had read about it in *Libelle* (*a women's magazine in The Netherlands*) but that article was about hypnosis. So it was something completely different. Really a coincidence.

Th. Well, we will have to send *Libelle* a flower then won't we? But let us temper our optimism a little bit.

C. Even if it was again as when we were married.

H. Yes, right.

Again an episode whereby the therapist assesses the client's motivation. His last remark indicates that he understands and is empathic.

Th. Are you a person that sticks to agreements whatever it may cost?

C. Yes.

Th. That is what I thought.

Here the therapist is being empathic and understanding.

Th. You have had several forms of treatment, haven't you and once a fortnight in a clinic?

C. (*Gets upset*)

Th. You are a little . . . you get upset easily, don't you, you cry easily. Is that your mood during these last days or is it because we are talking about it?

C. The last couple of weeks.

Th. You are really at the end of your tether.

C. Yes, now and then you would quit.

Th. Yes, I understand.

C. Last week I had the urge to tear the drinking fountain off the wall.

Th. I can really understand that, it feels if there is no way out.

C. Yes.

Th. And then we also made you wait for a couple of weeks.

The therapist is empathic and is showing his expertise and knowledge. He is predicting the symptom-free part of her life.

Th. Do you experience any pleasure in things?

C. Yes, if I know that I am leaving.

Th. You mean if everything is alright, everything has been checked?

C. Yes.

Th. And outside of your home you are rid of everything for a while?

C. Yes.

He provides the husband with important information regarding his wife's condition and the prevalence of the symptoms.

H.   Does this illness occur often?

Th. Well, hard to say. In your home town, there are about 30 to 40 people who have had the same diagnosis during the past year.

Here the therapist is quite directive and offers advice. He actually tells the husband not to sell his house and move because of his wife's symptoms.

H.   Well, I have been thinking about what I could do to help. Maybe sell the house and move back to where our relatives live?!

Th. No, you should wait till after the treatment. Then you can decide. In fact I would not advise you to take such measures on the basis of your wife's complaints. The important thing is, it is not the surroundings that cause these problems. Your wife should get control back over everything. As soon as she has mastered that, you can freely decide where and how to live.

H.   Yes, because living here is more expensive and there is always the possibility that here she will keep her problem.

Th. Right, moving never is a solution.

H.   Right.

Th. Now, let us first see how your wife responds to therapy.

It is important here, more explicitly than anywhere else in this conversation, that the therapist explains what the treatment programme entails, the rationale for the therapeutic procedures and the necessity for the client's co-operation. Again this is an assessment of her motivation for therapy.

Th. The therapeutic programme is tailored to get you again to do things without repeating or checking. Eventually your checking will disappear completely. In this way your self-confidence which is now very low will return. This will happen step by step and in a way that you will agree with. There is no forcing things, step by step. The programme consists of four parts. During the first month you will monitor and record what you do and how often you do so. In this way we will have an idea of the state of affairs right now. This takes four weeks. Then, the most important part of the programme begins. It is called exposure and consists of four weeks with twice weekly one hour sessions. In between the sessions there are tasks that you have to do yourself at home. These tasks all have to do with compulsions. This means doing some things without repetition or checking. In the beginning these tasks are quite easy but they will become increasingly more difficult. They will eventually become very tough. Initially, we need to agree which steps you will take. They will become very difficult for you, but remember never too difficult. Beforehand we agree upon the steps that you take, increasingly they will be more difficult, which I know will become a very hard time for you.

The therapist emphasizes the tailor-made aspect of the programme and the self-control procedure. Again his expertise and knowledge is emphasized.

Th. What it is all about is that you learn to tolerate the fear and anxiety, and to experience that not giving in to the compulsion will, in the end, lead to a decrease in anxiety. Nowadays, you never reach this point because you always give in to the compulsion. Not giving in will first lead to higher anxiety, tension increases, but then it will slowly disappear and will never reach the top again. That is what we are going to teach you, first with little things.

This section contains an informative element, an assessment of motivation and instills some hope.

Th. I have said something about improvement. You should be able to function normally and without me, but you will have your little worry now and then but never to the extent that you really are in trouble again. That is the goal that we want to reach and that is not nothing. So keep this in mind during the inevitable difficult moments during the coming months. It is not for nothing, keep in mind that now you are sweating for your health.

We will now turn to strategies designed to maintain a collaborative set by encouraging active participation, by exerting pressure, by mobilizing social support, by promoting the treatment and its procedures, by providing support and by helping, i.e., by making the problems more manageable, and by suggesting ways to handle these.

5　Maintaining a collaborative set

Introduction

Once a client has engaged in the treatment process, it then is necessary to establish a collaborative set. A collaborative set is the aspect of the therapeutic relationship in which the therapist encourages the client to relinquish old habits and experiment with new behaviours, cognitions and attitudes. This set has a particular effect on the therapeutic relationship, and enables the client to change within the context of a perceived positive relationship.

In a medical setting, changing the treatment setting as a way of enhancing compliance involves both "tailoring" and "convenience". *Convenience* programs focus on a group of clients that are in treatment in a particular setting. One tries to make this setting as accessible and as simple as possible. Attempts are made to limit the waiting periods; clients see the same doctor and nurse each time; they can visit the doctor on demand and the pharmacy is near by, always having the prescribed medication available. *Tailoring* is a process that adapts the treatment as much as possible to the client's individual life style and habits.

Therapists can also introduce changes in their own practice. Many therapists do not have a separate filing system for particular clients defined by diagnosis. They could for example reorganize client files so that they can get a clearer overview of their policy towards types of clients. It is possible to monitor the treatment and the next appointment using a special filing system or computer program. In this way, missed appointments will be noticed and the client can be followed up. Generally, giving information to clients about their disorder, possible consequences, existing treatment and the side-effects of medication is considered essential in order to gain clients' co-operation. It is also clear that information alone has little impact on changing life style and in some circumstances may even decrease compliance. Attempts should be made to increase the clients' sense of responsibility through involving them more actively in the entire treatment program, e.g., by encouraging self-regulation of symptoms or other behaviours that are important for treatment.

The facilitating or inhibiting influence of the social environment on clients' health behaviour is now well recognized (Becker & Green, 1975). Sometimes clients may be encouraged not to comply with the prescriptions, possibly because family members find the regime is rather cumbersome and awkward. The client also does not look particularly ill and often does not understand the reason for the treatment. It may be helpful to involve one or more family members in the client's treatment, pointing out the importance of his or her support. The client can be helped in keeping appointments, taking medication or following homework instructions. It is important that this support does not have a belittling or punitive effect.

Clients can profit from such an approach even though the entire treatment program may not be intrinsically rewarding. Maintenance behaviour will not always result in noticeable changes, and extrinsically motivating strategies will sometimes have to be used.

The strategies described here have been developed to increase the cooperation of clients in medical settings but are also likely to be useful in psychotherapy. Some will be discussed and illustrated in this chapter, in which we focus specifically on establishing and maintaining the collaborative set. Compliance with treatment and responding to therapeutic initiatives depend on conveying to clients that the therapist is resourceful, trustworthy and capable of joining them in effecting change.

Maintaining a collaborative set

A study classifying relationship enhancement strategies, described in Chapter 3, indicated that therapists considered the following strategies as being very similar: encouraging active participation, applying pressure and securing social support. These strategies all share one characteristic: the therapist tries to establish a working alliance by creating a situation in which the client feels motivated to participate more actively in the therapeutic procedures and maintain negotiated agreements.

Encouraging active participation

A great number of studies have been conducted in attempts to unravel the relationship between therapeutic outcome and client characteristics. Some of these studies are essentially sociodemographic and have been reviewed elsewhere (e.g., Garfield & Bergin, 1986). More interesting for our discussion on motivating strategies are studies on process characteristics and outcome. Clients' behaviour in therapy may be thought of in terms of task behaviour and interpersonal behaviour. Relevant studies report evidence on the association of therapeutic outcome with the quantity and pattern of the clients' activity in therapy, such as speech and silence. Generally, these and similar studies seem to suggest that more active clients have a higher probability of successfully completing therapy with positive clinical outcomes (see, for example, Garfield & Bergin, 1986). Particularly important in this respect are self-control procedures such as the contingency contracting approach. We will illustrate this approach with a client who has, amongst other problems, difficulty studying.

Mr Latimer is in his late twenties. He leads a chaotic life and describes a social phobia in that when he is with other people he is constantly thinking about what they will think of him. As a result he spends days preparing for an encounter, rehearsing what he will say and inevitably fails in his endeavours. He has had a number of short-lived relationships and now has a LAT (living apart together) relationship with a nurse. He recognizes his need for perfection and terminated his academic studies when he had to write a paper on an extremely difficult assignment and was concerned about what his professor would think. His life is characterized by passive avoidance. The therapist and Mr Latimer decided to focus on the paper as a first treatment goal. The initial strategy was to monitor the amount of time he worked on the paper. The first step in the actual construction of the paper was the collection of relevant literature. He had to find an article, book or chapter that looked like what he was planning and use it as a guide. He then made a list of subjects that could serve as chapter subsections and formulated a contract about writing it. He then had to write at least five lines, but also to agree on a penalty for not fulfilling his part of the "contract".

In this way, a model was presented about how to handle a larger problem and, in the longer term, other important aspects of his life. After the paper was successfully finished, which considerably increased his self-esteem, the social phobia was treated in a similar way, using small steps and formulating contingencies.

In cases like these, not completing the contract is often a problem. This may sometimes be addressed by introducing a particular consequence for the failure. This is illustrated in the following case of a therapist in therapy as part of his training.

The therapist has pointed out a number of problem areas that he would like to resolve during his treatment, including his problem with binge eating, which has resulted in a weight problem, as well as his inability to manage his time. He decided to focus on his weight as the first target for his self-control therapy. He was instructed to find out the caloric value of everything he ate and to record it for a month. During the next session, a month later, his mean daily intake was calculated to be 2900 calories, which was considered to be appropriate for the time being. If he consumed more than 2900 calories in any one day, he was to wake up earlier than usual the next day and run a fixed number of miles depending on the excess calories from the previous day. At this point in treatment, the therapist expressed his concern about not being able to get out of bed that early. Together with his wife, he was asked about what the consequence should be if he did not go jogging after a day of excessive eating. They decided on a task that he always avoided (in this case, doing the laundry). Not surprisingly, he did not have to do the laundry since he stuck with the treatment program. The program led to considerable weight loss. Attention was directed to his problems in organizing his schedule through time management.

Sometimes clients can be encouraged to co-operate using more simple strategies.

Ms Patterson is an 18-year-old young woman presenting with a borderline personality disorder but who has also a well-developed sense of humour. It was obvious that she would establish a good therapeutic relationship through which a self-control procedure for her self-mutilation could be developed. She was confronted with the choice between being diagnosed as having a mental health problem with a poor prognosis or as a developmental disorder with a better prognosis. She insisted that she was not insane and chose to actively participate in a self-control treatment program. She was able to get rid of her automutilation habit with the self-control procedure within the scheduled 13 weeks.

All of these cases share the feature that the therapist more or less explicitly asks the client to co-operate. Of course, clients accept or decline this, but all decisions need to be made on the basis of the client's own choice in an atmosphere of negotiation. In contrast to this approach, a series of strategies can be used by therapists that result in a more cooperative client attitude, using different forms of pressure. It should be kept in mind, that each of these are ways that the therapist can keep the client engaged, show the value of treatment and maintain the collaborative set.

Exerting pressure

Mr Robertson, who had a long history of drug dependence, wanted to stop his life of managing his daily heroin fix. He had an unkempt appearance, was dishevelled and wore dirty clothes. Instead of beginning immediately with a therapeutic program, the therapist asked him what he was prepared to invest in his treatment, in other words, how important did he feel overcoming his dependence was to him. The therapist then went on to ask if he was prepared to change his appearance completely, to wear clean presentable clothing and have a haircut as an indication of his commitment to treatment. After some negotiation, the client made these outward changes and treatment eventually started with success. Apart from the fact that this intervention forced the client to consider carefully his commitment and motivation, it effectively prevented him from returning to the drug scene, where his new "outfit" would have caused considerable embarrassment.

Therapists may also exert pressure by linking clinical progress to therapeutic time and investment. In fact, therapeutic change can sometimes be achieved by negotiating the therapeutic hour, as is illustrated in the following case.

Mr Rose, a 27-year-old intelligent client with a speech and hearing handicap, requested help because of his obsessive-compulsive problems. He had developed a very complicated system of compulsions, some of which involved his parents. For example, when he went to the bathroom his parents had to perform particular rituals such as walking back and forth in front of the opened bathroom door before he could leave. This obviously caused a great deal of strain and inconvenience. The first six sessions were used to track his complicated compulsions and to develop clear communication between him and the therapist. The sessions progressed slowly because of the strained communication. Fortunately, the therapist was patient and gave him the time he needed, which proved to be the basis of a good therapeutic relationship. However, as a consequence of this, the client felt at ease in the session and progress was very slow indeed, which was distressing for his parents. It was decided to increase both pace and pressure. One of the problems during the first phase of treatment was that Mr Rose did not carry out contingencies that were agreed upon. He had to "pay" in terms of writing and reading assignments, and carry out household chores. He always found reasons that subtly changed the agreed contract. The only task that was completed reasonably well was his writing in a diary about his life as a handicapped person, which was a first step in exerting more pressure. An intervention that was considered by the therapist, and which had worked well with other clients, was that Mr Rose would have to call the therapist if he had failed on an assignment. The therapist predicted that he would not fail, but because of his speech handicap this could not be implemented. It was also assumed that since the therapeutic relationship was extremely important to him, he would consider the therapist an important and attractive person, and that an alternative was that the duration of the session could be part of the contract. Therapy time should be "earned', so that not maintaining the contract would lead to shorter sessions. Following this strategy, the treatment went much more smoothly and his parents' neutralizing activity could cease, much to their relief. Progress continued steadily from this point in time.

Some clients, as may have been the case with Mr Rose, use the therapeutic session to neutralize feelings of tension and anxiety, so that pressure to change can be increased by limiting the amount of time the therapist makes available.

Perhaps the situation that best illustrates the principle of exerting pressure is the self-control treatment of disturbances of impulse control. This approach can be seen as spinning a web of pressure. We will illustrate this approach with two cases: a client with pathological gambling habits and another with frequent outbursts of aggression.

Mr Yates is a 44-year-old shopkeeper who has built up considerable debt because of his frequent visits to the casino. The following sequence emerged following his assessment: tension → thoughts about gambling → decision to go to the casino → arrange for money → drive towards the casino → enter the casino → sit at the table → play → feelings of guilt after gambling → increased tension. The interventions directed towards each of these phases included:

1   Reducing tension using relaxation exercises (progressive relaxation), alternative relaxing activities (his hobby), immediate motor activities (e.g., running).
2   Monitoring his gambling thoughts and undertaking household chores or his carpentry hobby.
3   Once having made the decision to go to the casino, he should phone his wife and tell her about his plans. She should not reason, but should arrange for him to have access to an already determined sum of money.
4   He should not take the shortest route to the casino; but should follow an alternative, longer one.
5   When at the casino, he should not be allowed to enter immediately, but should go back to his car and think things over for a fixed amount of time.
6   When he does play, the amount of time is fixed. And if he does not keep the agreement, he is to do all household activities for one week. He has to alternate between playing for 15 minutes and watching for 15 minutes.
7   All winnings are given to his wife and she should choose how it is spent.
8   Eventually he may only play roulette and not his preferred game of blackjack. Each time a step is added that makes gambling more awkward and less attractive.
9   After his visit to the casino he is to "pay" his wife in the form of household activities.
10   Any break in the chain of events results in a fixed amount of money to be put aside and used for a holiday.

The important intervention in this case was the fact that Mr Yates' wife was mobilized in the treatment. This increased the pressure to stick to the agreements and eventually to break his habit and work through the stressors controlling his habits. A similar approach was used with Mr Williams' aggressive bouts.

Mr Williams is a 39-year-old bricklayer living on a government disability allowance. His wife holds a job outside the house for 4 days a week. His complaint is that he often feels very tense and is easily irritated. He quickly looses control of his aggression and looses his temper, which is usually followed by an aggressive outburst. The situations that trigger his aggression can be anything, like a barking dog or his wife not acknowledging him for doing housework. He has, on occasions, been violent, but his wife has succeeded in preventing injury. After such episodes he is full of regret, though it usually takes a couple of days before he is able to apologize to his wife. Their marital relationship is reasonably satisfactory, but his self-esteem is very low. The first therapeutic intervention consisted of encouraging Mr Williams to start some meaningful work such as model building or youth work. When he felt tense, he was to do motor activities such as cycling, walking or relaxation exercises. During the sessions the frustrations were expired, and the therapist tried to change his view of the situation and his behaviour through role playing and humour. The high-risk situations were considered and appropriate coping skills were developed. Since Mr Williams got very tense before an aggressive outburst, his tension was explicitly described in terms of physical symptoms and used as a cue to leave the situation. If an aggressive bout occurred, he was to apologize, repair the damage or do something which was disliked. After five sessions, Mr Williams reported that he was in better control of his aggression and, even though no outburst had occurred, he reported having used the interventions and relaxation exercises whenever he felt tense.

Mobilizing social support

Although human communication and interaction within families is less positive and polite than between relative strangers, some positive interchanges are necessary in all interactions. Emotional support in an intimate relationship is necessary in maintaining the psychological, and even physical, well-being of family members, probably through its positive effect on everyone's self-esteem. This support, expressed, in part by positive and non-aversive interactions, functions as a kind of buffer against the damaging effects of negative life events and other problems.

The literature on Expressed Emotion (EE), in the context of psychiatric disorders, presents some evidence in support of the relationship between negative communication and psychological distress (see Falloon et al., 1984). Increased critical and hostile remarks, along with expressions of emotional overinvolvement, increase the probability of symptomatic relapse. It has also been shown that clients from high-EE and low-EE families do not differ in degree of pathology at intake or discharge. Differences have, therefore, to be present in the families and in their reaction towards the client. These differences do seem to reflect levels of tolerance, attitudes towards the acceptance of the disorder and coping style.

During the 1960s some therapeutic approaches emphasized the pathogenic aspect of family interaction. It was assumed that psychopathology was the outcome of negative family interaction. This point of view has been questioned and, more recently, the stress–vulnerability hypothesis has been considered the best explanation for the relationship between psychopathology and family interaction. These ideas have resulted in the development of a psychosocial approach towards family interaction and family therapy in differing psychiatric disorders. There is also considerable evidence to reject the idea that pathological families *per se* can lead to a range of psychological disorders. This can be illustrated through the well-documented case of agoraphobia described by Arrindell and Emmelkamp (1985). They reported that spouses of agoraphobic clients did not report more complaints than spouses in a control group. Moreover, agoraphobic women experienced their marital relationship as less distressing than did women with other psychiatric complaints. These results do not support the hypothesis that complaints such as agoraphobia are a function of the relationship. Moreover, marital therapy for agoraphobia, although leading towards an improvement in the relationship, does not reduce the avoidance behaviour, whereas exposure reduces complaints in both the relationship and agoraphobia. There is also evidence that involving the spouse in individual therapy for a panic disorder with agoraphobia will lead to better results.

It may be concluded that, where possible, spouses should be involved in the treatments that use exposure, as this may lead to a reduction in complaints and an improved marital relationship. In these cases, spouse-aided therapy would be sufficient. Sometimes the treatment of agoraphobia is successful but the existing marital problems still remain. Here it would be easier to change the focus to marital therapy, and the risk of relapse would be reduced. Where marital problems are so distressing that they prevent the treatment of the agoraphobia, marital therapy could be offered and individual treatment could be delayed. The same approach could be used for the treatment of other disorders suggesting that making appropriate use of social support is important in treatment (Bennun & Schindler, 1988).

Ms Simpson is a 45-year-old housewife with an obsessive-compulsive disorder. She is insecure about not having heard things correctly and neutralizes her fear by wishing everybody well, by touching things and by asking her husband for reassurance. In the first phase of treatment, and after she began self-monitoring, an attempt was made to stop her husband's reinforcing activity. Mr Simpson was also asked to consider making their life more positive by going out together and doing things that they both enjoyed. He even was moved to be nice and thoughtful to her if she was not questioning him (i.e., showing her rituals). However, this proved not to be successful because she forced her husband to answer her questions, sometimes after 7 hours of questioning, yelling at him and/or having a panic attack. During the next session her behaviour was labeled positively as a sign of her strong personality but was also labeled negatively as behaving like a little child with her father. It was obvious that stopping her husband's response was too great a step. She was asked if she could wait for just one minute before her husband answered her neutralizing question. She indicated that she could, and it was agreed that he would also wait a minute, and if she still wished, he would then answer her queries. Moreover, it was suggested that obsessions do not disappear spontaneously: every obsession that disappears has been "thought out" of her mind.

These attempts to mobilize social support might even go further, as was the case with Mrs Tucker.

Mrs Tucker is the wife of a client with a compulsive personality disorder. She experiences, understandably, a lot of strain having to live with a man who requests that everything be "in order". They also have a 2-year-old son, making it impossible to make their lives predictable and perfect. Her treatment comprised of stress management and coaching in a response cost procedure.

A stress management program was started in which Mrs Tucker coupled increasingly unpleasant physical sensations of tension to more invasive coping techniques, varying from breathing exercises to time-out procedures. The most extreme intervention consisted of packing her suitcase, picking up her son and going to her parents who lived close by. This would happen with her husband's cooperation, who agreed that his behaviour was extreme and who acknowledged her plight. The next phase addressed her husband's personality difficult. Using exposure and response prevention for obsessive-compulsive symptoms, particular rooms in their house were indicated as "common" or "shared" rooms, i.e., they were not be contaminated with his problematic personality. He was to refrain from making any comments about cleanliness and order, and agreed to pay a small amount of money each time he broke the agreement. Mrs Tucker would then be able to spend this money any way she wished, and this, together with similar interventions, led to a reasonably manageable relationship as well as a life without too much strain, enabling Mr Tucker to engage in his own therapy. Obviously, arrangements like these will only work when things happen in a supportive atmosphere which, for persons with personalities like Mr Tucker's, is not always easy to make happen.

Helping with the process of change

Strupp (1978), defined psychotherapy as an interpersonal process designed to bring about modifications of feelings, cognitions, attitudes and behaviour which have proved troublesome to the person seeking help from a trained professional. Psychotherapy, therefore, is concerned with personality and behaviour change. Clients who seek help for psychological problems desire change—they want to feel or act differently, and the therapist agrees to assist them in achieving this goal. The process of therapy is designed not to change clients but to help them change themselves (Strupp, 1978). The important question, then, is how is this achieved? All schools of psychotherapy have tried to answer this question but, as described in Chapter 2, some general directions can be formulated that point to the common features of the healing situation. In this section we will focus on motivating strategies that are derived from the helping process itself as a way of maintaining the collaborative set.

Promoting the treatment

One could define *promoting the treatment* as the therapist adapting therapeutic plans and their presentation to match the client's needs and preferences.

Since rational discussion is an important ingredient of psychotherapy, it is necessary that therapists are aware of findings from social psychological research on persuasion and attitude change (McGuire, 1985). Any change of opinion in the desired direction is more likely if the speaker is considered credible on the basis of knowledge and trustworthiness. This influence is stronger, immediately after the message rather than following a delay, and the effectiveness of a message increases if the speaker begins with opinions that are shared by the listener. Moreover, such speaker characteristics as race and religion, which have nothing to do with the particular discussion, can strongly influence acceptance. Furthermore, ways of uncovering feelings of fear are only effective, in so far as they also offer concrete advice. Any indication that attempts are being made to manipulate the listener will increase resistance and opposition, whereas humour will decrease this resistance. Finally, successful persuasion is not only targeted towards the attitudes themselves, but particularly to the reasons the listener has for having a particular attitude. It is important to be aware of these results when considering those motivating strategies that are based on the client's interactional style, since this usually will reflect their needs and preferences.

Ms Campbell is a 40-year-old housewife suffering from primary obsessional slowness. Because she conducts her rituals in such a slow and deliberate way, she makes no mistakes, and she therefore experiences little tension and anxiety. The compulsion sequence is as follows: "Help, I did something wrong" → anxiety and tension → neutralizing activities, checking, repetitions. Two mechanisms play an important role in this case. First, there is extreme avoidance of doing anything that might trigger tension and anxiety; and secondly, her behaviour can be seen as small steps that are carried out piece by piece. An activity is first "thought out" completely then repeated in her mind, and then carried out. Every step in the chain is slow and meticulous and, like other slow clients, Ms Campbell succeeds in experiencing relatively little tension and anxiety. Any treatment is considered as threatening, since her way of doing things will be fundamentally altered.

Motivating these clients for treatment is a long process and a crucial step in helping them is making a distinction between short-term and long-term problems, and short-term and long-term solutions. In other words, a long-term solution is best achieved by short-term suffering and distress.

For other clients, the therapist's motivational activity is more explicitly tailored to their personal needs.

Mr Leicester experienced great difficulties following his wife's extramarital affair and her unsuccessful marital therapy. During the intake procedure he demanded contact with someone from the helping profession and managed to disrupt the counselling centre. During the intake session his communication was incoherent and he said that he was unable to understand the interviewer. When he was asked, he did not follow but continued in his unclear, disqualifying manner. Later in therapy, the therapist found out that he used this way of relating to others in order to avoid change. It seemed as if he wanted to demonstrate that, although he had a lot of problems completing his education, he nevertheless was an intelligent and subtle person. The therapist gained the impression that Mr Leicester wanted to show the therapist as being capable, while at the same time show that he was superior to the therapist. It was clear to the therapist and supervisor that Mr Leicester would have to change his goals if he was to achieve anything in therapy. It was decided that the therapist would begin by offering Mr Leicester what he wanted, i.e., help in managing his pain about his wife hurting him through the extramarital affair. He also treated Mr Leicester with respect since he did not want to antagonize him, and did so by asking him for his view on matters, but at the same time remained concrete. The therapist did not refrain from confrontation, but only allowed confrontation after a good relationship had been established so that Mr Leicester had sufficient time during the session to digest the messages about the value of treatment.

Providing support

Support by the therapist can be defined as the therapist's strengthening the client's self-confidence. All interventions that increase the client's self-esteem are included in this general heading. Therapists' support should be distinguished from all interventions designed to initiate or mobilize the support of the social environment from the therapist.

Mr and Mrs Jones both live on a government allowance. Mrs Jones is a manic depressive client who is reasonably stable but has had a number of psychotic episodes. Mr Jones has an obsessive-compulsive disorder and continually checks with his fingers. The chain of activities usually ends when he prepares a drink or a meal. During these activities, the two do not speak to each other, as this would disturb his rhythm and cause a repetition of the sequence. His wife may interrupt the sequence by suggesting a walk. It is during these moments that he is symptom-free, but he is not able to do other enjoyable things, such as listening to music. There is a strong relational component to the problem because Mrs Jones is worried, but not particularly worried that her husband has this complaint; moreover, the couple did not request therapy but just accepted their "illness". Since both partners are on a government allowance and any improvement could result in a loss of income, the therapist chose to reassure them. He did not offer them therapy as such, but rather his advice was to accept and adapt to their situation. He gave them the usual exposure and response prevention program. The husband was asked to monitor each day the way he accepted his condition. To assist him in this acceptance he was advised to go out for a walk with his wife for 2 hours each day. Walking was linked to improvement and acceptance of his condition. This procedure led to a decrease in compulsive behaviour and improved self-esteem.

Ms MacDonald is a 34-year-old, married mother with four children presenting with complex symptomatology: dysmorphophobia, panic disorder with agoraphobia, depression and alcohol problems. She also has sensitive traits and is passive–aggressive. Since Ms MacDonald is a very creative person (with talent and interest in music, painting, poetry), it was decided that art should be the avenue for change. The therapist described her as a person with a broken heart and whose soul was wounded. The therapeutic program consisted of a "balanced menu" of art and rest, with some success.

Offering help

Helping is different from support. The therapist assists the client in making the presenting problems manageable and suggests ways in which these can be carried out adequately. In a sense the therapist does the things that the client is unable to do. This implies that the outcome of the assessment phase of treatment can, in itself, constitute a crucial motivational step.

Ms Sharpe is a client with alcohol problems and who has suffered pathological grief since her husband, who she idealized, left the marriage. The therapist relabeled her condition and told her that her problems were caused by the fact that both positive and negative feelings were becoming confused. He advised her to disentangle her feelings by using a diary and write out on the left side the positive feelings and on the right side her negative feelings. As a result of this minimal intervention, she improved considerably. Next, the alcohol abuse problem was treated with a self-control procedure.

Annette is a 16-year-old girl with panic attacks. She had received three sessions with hyperventilation provocation that successfully reduced her panic attacks. Her parents felt that she should be more adult, but she was reluctant to change. When her parents arranged a holiday for her and a male friend, she then started to have panic attacks again. Her attacks were reinterpreted as a transition problem on her road to adulthood. She was advised to imitate a hyperventilation attack each time she wanted or needed affection or attention from her mother. The rationale was as follows: your complaints give you attention from your mother. You do not have to wait for that, you can get that anytime you want. This advice resulted in her asking for attention in a more appropriate way.

The following vignette highlights a number of the motivating strategies presented in this chapter.

A verbatim illustration of motivating strategies to maintain the collaborative set

Mr Strong is a 20-year-old unemployed carpenter. He was referred to the outpatient clinic following episodes of exhibitionism. He is from a very deprived background and was sexually abused at a very young age. Although he is physically an attractive young man, he has great difficulty expressing himself. He has exposed himself about once a fortnight, over a period of 10 years. This problem has brought him in contact with the police on a number of occasions. He appears highly motivated to change his habit, but years of client-centered therapy did not bring about any noticeable change. This vignette is from the fourth session.

The therapist is being empathic by discussing two topics that were introduced by the client in the preceding session: his new outfit and relationships.

Th. Hello Mike! Take the seat . . . How was Christmas? . . . I bet you looked smashing in your new outfit.

C. Yes, well . . . I think . . . I told you . . . I went to this shop with my sister . . . I wanted to look nice . . . for Christmas you know . . . and bought this tuxedo and tie . . . Really nice.

Th. Any success with the girls, Mike?

C. (smiles) Well, at least . . . I felt good in the outfit . . . we had a reasonable time at Christmas . . . at home first . . . that was not really fun . . . then in my sister's home . . . she's married . . . that was nice . . . Dinner and so on . . . and then I went out with my mother's boyfriend . . . we went to this pub . . . it wasn't bad!

The therapist is applying pressure by talking about the agreement that was made during the previous session.

Th. Could you please repeat the deal that we made about your exposing yourself, just to make sure that we understand each other.

C. Yes . . . if I cannot resist . . . the urge . . . and expose myself . . . then I have to walk for two hours . . . to the next city.

The therapist is being caring, thereby increasing his attractiveness. He is also increasing the pressure by challenging the client, suggesting that the client is unable to keep to the agreement.

Th. And you're allowed to take the train back . . . Yeah, I worried about that. Can you keep that up for two hours. That's an awful long time! Your feet will be full of blisters.

C. No problem . . . I can manage that . . . I have done that before.

Th. So, next time we can make the deal that you go back on foot and leave the train?! (smiles)

C. Well . . . I don't know about that . . . not just now . . . I will have to go into training.

Th. You're really a sportsman, aren't you? Running and swimming. And always on your bike.

C. Yeah . . . can't afford a car (smiles).

The therapist is supporting the client by positively labeling any relapse. He is also exploring the problem and describing it in resolvable terms.

Th. We haven't seen each other for . . . well . . . three weeks. . . Christmas and holidays. Did you have to do the running? I hope you had to because it would indicate that you are someone that sticks to his agreements.

C. No . . . I didn't have to . . . I have felt the urge twice though . . . but I fought it.

Th. Well done! Could you describe what happened?

C. The first was . . . right after I left the office . . . after our last talk . . . I felt tense and excited . . . It has happened before.

Th. You mean that you find these sessions a strain and difficult, that is a good sign . . . it means that you are working at your therapy . . . it is not something that leaves you unaffected . . . and tension is channelled into excitement. We will have to do something about that.

Here again the therapist is empathic and helping the client in managing his problems and handling them appropriately. He is providing explanations for the presenting behaviour.

C. The second time . . . eh . . . was when I went out . . . a couple of weeks ago . . . I go to this pub with my mother's . . . eh . . . boyfriend. He is the only person I go out with. And I . . . ehm . . . sometimes get bored . . . then I see all these couples in the pub enjoying themselves . . . and the girls . . . and then after the pub closes . . . I walk towards the park . . . and the excitement increases.

Th. But this time you fought the urge successfully.

C. Yeah . . . I went home . . . and read something.

Th. Good! Well done! . . . I was thinking about how we can handle the tension. What about your sexual excitement . . . did you masturbate?

C. Yeah, I jacked off . . . and that somewhat . . . eased the tension.

Th. I think that's a sensible thing to do . . . do you feel guilty or childish about it?

C. No . . . not really . . . but I feel lonely.

Th. That's the next step to overcome your loneliness . . . let's solve the problems in the right order.

The therapist continues helping the client to overcome his problem. He signals his problem with assertiveness and dating, and introduces a stress management program where interventions are formulated for increasing levels of tension.

Th. Let's try and see how things are connected . . . let's see . . . you are in a situation where you do not really feel at ease . . . here in therapy because you have to talk about yourself . . . in the pub because you rather go out with someone else than your mother's boyfriend.

C.   You can say that again.

Th. You'd rather have a girlfriend or friends . . . in short, you feel lonely.

C.   Yeah.

Th. Then the tension increases.

C.   Yeah.

Th. It is important that later on we try and describe how you experience this tension because we will have to consider that as a cue to do something about.

C.   Uhm . . . How do you mean?

Th. Well, for instance, when you get tense you may feel something in your stomach.

C.   Right . . . a kind of . . . ehm . . . spasm.

Th. You could consider this spasm as a signal to do something about the tension.

C.   Like . . . you mean . . . relaxing.

Th. Yes, do something that will make you feel relaxed . . . concentrate on your body, relax your stomach muscles, go to the bathroom and try and relax there or even go out, put on your running shoes and run! Later on we will construct a program for that.

The therapist is increasing the pressure by showing that he is not satisfied with a simple yes or no. The atmosphere is clearly supportive and positive.

C.   I see.

Th. Do you really see? (*smiles*)

C.   (*smiles*) Yes, I understand . . . I really do.

The atmosphere continues to be positive and supportive. The therapist is still exerting pressure by discussing the time limitation and, the first agreement made in the intake session.

Th. Where were we? . . . we were trying to describe what happened when you feel tense . . . then when the pub closes you go out . . . do you go home?

C.   More or less . . . that direction . . . I go to the park . . . there is a student home . . . near the park

Th. The place where you call and expose yourself.

C.   Yes.

Th. What happens on the way . . . what are you saying to yourself? We will eventually have to get this whole chain . . . and as I explained before . . . at each link we will have to look for ways that increase the chance of breaking the chain.

C.   Yes I understand.

Th. And we have to reach our goal in a short time . . . in ten sessions we will have to reach our goal.

The therapist is showing his expertise by correctly formulating the therapeutic goal. He is implying that the exhibitionism is the result of a psychological problem, i.e., dealing with tension and, at a deeper level, overcoming fear of loss of face. The atmosphere is supportive using humour if appropriate.

Th. What is our goal?
C. The exposing.
Th. Or the tension and excitement?!
C. Because . . . they kind of trigger the exposing!
Th. Right . . . good student! (*smiles*)
C. (*smiles*)

The therapist is positively relabeling the client's problem while maintaining pressure to change.

Th. Okay, we keep our deal that you do the running when you cannot fight the urge . . . the running is important . . . it shows that you are prepared to work hard.

The therapist is promoting the treatment procedure (relaxation exercises) and providing a good rationale for it.

Th. What about the tension? Have you had any experience with relaxation exercises?
C. Yes . . . a couple of years ago.
Th. Did you work with a cassette?
C. No . . . no cassette . . . I would feel silly.
Th. Okay, the next session we will spend totally on relaxation exercises . . . and look and see how we can guarantee that you can fight the tension.

The therapist is maintaining the atmosphere of exploring change by attempting to increase self-esteem. He is also motivating the client to negotiate about the self-control procedures.

Th. I keep thinking about you as a sportsman . . . how can we use your athletic skills to counter tension? Have you ever thought about doing the triathlon . . . I mean you can run, you swim well, you ride your bike.
C. I have to.
Th. I know it's poverty that forces you (*smiles*).
C. (*smiles*) I also have . . . almost all . . . my diplomas for swimming instruction.
Th. Not bad!
C. I have been . . . thinking about going to the . . . ehm . . . swimming pool three times . . . per week and . . . get my last diplomas . . . that's what I would . . . love to do . . . being a swimming instructor.

Th. And you would be an excellent one I think.

C. And I have . . . also been thinking about . . . the triathlon.

The therapist is maintaining a working alliance by trying to develop some social support. In this case the client will have to build this up on his own. Sport is a good context for him to do so.

Th. Do you know anything about training schedules.

C. Well . . . I know this sports school . . . I could go and ask . . . perhaps there are other people . . . who want to train for the triathlon . . . it is better to do so in a group . . . you help each other in this way.

An appointment is made for the next session in 2 weeks' time and the client expresses his feeling that finally something pragmatic is being done about his complaint.

Th. Right . . . well . . . let's see . . . we already have a whole list of agreements and deals . . . you run for two hours if you expose . . . you are allowed to take the train back . . . next time you will have to run or walk back (*smiles*) then you go to this sports school and get the information you need . . . there probably is also a triathlon association as part of the Athletic Association . . . perhaps you could phone them or write them.

C. No . . . I will . . . ehm . . . phone them.

Th. You find that difficult? . . . to pick up the phone and talk to them?

C. No I have . . . done that before . . . they are there to answer.

Th. And you ask in the sports school if there are any others who are in training for the triathlon?

C. Yes.

Th. Do we have to formulate consequences in case you are not able to go there or to phone?

C. No . . . I'll go . . . guaranteed.

Th. And you will go to the swimming pool three times each week? When?

C. I will do so . . . three days will be alright.

Th. You will have to do more running if you are not going to swim! (*smiles*)

C. (*smiles*) I know.

Conclusions

This short vignette illustrates some of the strategies therapists can use in their attempts to maintain a working collaborative set. It is important that the client experiences the therapist as someone thinking *with* them about change and offering help and support in bringing about changes in what presents as distressing complaints. By showing that they have the expertise to suggest new ways to deal with problematic situations, the therapist can vary the amount of pressure they exert in encouraging the client to try out alternative behaviours and maintain therapeutic agreements. The social psychology literature on persuasion that we examined earlier indicates some of the avenues that can be explored in enhancing the attraction of the therapeutic relationship and its effectiveness in bringing about change. Each client must obviously be viewed as a single case and the various elements outlined in these chapters can be used as clients and situations dictate.

Part III
RESEARCH IMPLICATIONS

In Part III we focus on the state of the art of research. Chapter 6 is devoted to methodological problems in psychotherapy research. Chapter 7 presents a selective overview of research conducted in the field thus far. We conclude finally with a description and discussion of a quasi-experimental study on the effect of enhancing the quality of the therapeutic relationship. The challenge for further research is to formulate and test additional strategies for handling problematic situations in the therapeutic relationship. Furthermore, indications are needed for the use of these strategies according to the demands of situational or client behaviour characteristics, as indicated from this review.

6 Methodological considerations

Introduction

In order to gain more empirical knowledge about strategies of social influence and their impact within the different phases of the therapeutic interaction, the actual process of change within and across therapy sessions needs to be studied. This study is called *process research* and is defined as the analysis of the interaction between the systems of the therapist and the client. It is the aim of this type of research to identify the process of change within the client-therapist interaction. The object of study encompasses the behaviour and experiences of both client and therapist in an attempt to identify the change process within and between sessions (Greenberg & Pinsof, 1986). The social interaction between client and therapist is one focus of process research. Its role is important since within the sessions, changes occur and conditions are created to change the client's everyday situation.

Intervention techniques, such as relaxation training or exposure, are of lesser interest, since a great deal is already known about the way they work; less is known, however, about what actually happens during a session. It is both the techniques and the conversation that form the basis of psychological treatment, and it is through the medium of conversation that motivation is increased, the treatment rationale is explained and resistance is tackled. In Chapter 2, these aspects were described as part of social influence. Whereas the intervention techniques in behaviour therapy are empirically based, this is not the case for the conversational elements. Furthermore, while it is necessary to maintain client motivation, it is less clear how this is achieved with a wide range of clients.

Although process research has a 30-year history, the basic experimental paradigm has essentially remained the same over this period. Research on therapy has been primarily concerned with showing the effectiveness of one school of psychotherapy, or one single intervention, whereas individual initiatives have been reported that include aspects of the therapeutic relationship and its impact on therapeutic success. Most of these research endeavours are limited to studying therapist and client personality characteristics and correlating these with outcome. The style of therapy as a stable behavioural tendency has been studied by clients rating therapist behaviour on a global measure immediately after the session. Sometimes independent observers judge sections from separate sessions using rating scales and infer global characteristics.

Some studies conducted within behavioural therapy have demonstrated that the quality of the therapeutic relationship influences outcome. Particular dimensions of therapist behaviour can be studied; these are of importance in so far as they affect clients' experience and facilitate positive outcomes. Indeed, studies that have investigated stable characteristics or styles have justifiably been the subject of much criticism (Fiske, 1977; Johnson & Matross, 1977; Parloff et al, 1978). Personality characteristics only allow for indirect inference about the behaviour shown in different stages of therapy and with different abstraction, they do not describe behaviours in different contexts. As Fiske (1977) emphasized, it makes little sense to study constructs that are apparently reflected in concrete behaviour, if they can be studied much more appropriately in another way.

If the mechanisms of social change are to be studied systematically, this implies that an analysis must be done on what transpires in different sessions, i.e., an analysis on the level of behaviours. In such an endeavour, the question arises as to what units of conversation can be described that enable a particular client to benefit from particular influences at a particular point in time (Kiesler, 1971; Zimmer, 1983). In this way, well-defined units of therapist behaviour can be selected as independent variables, and the behaviour and the client as dependent variables.

The first attempts at differentiating the therapeutic process into these units of observation and constructing a model of therapeutic influence, have been described as the first-generation process analysis (Auld & Whyte, 1959; Snyder, 1945; Strupp, 1955). In these early studies, large samples of audio-taped therapy sessions were coded and the data were then analysed sequentially. In the 1960s, the qualitative analysis of stylistic aspects of therapy was influenced by the research tradition in client-centred therapies. A decade later and within a new tradition, the limitations of the early studies (such as sampling problems, the use of different instruments and a focus on different complex levels) were overcome (e.g., Hill, 1978).

A conceptual framework for the analysis of social interaction during therapy

Greenberg (1986a) and Greenberg and Pinsof (1986) formulated a conceptual framework that systematized and coordinated process research. Different hierarchically ordered levels of what occurs within a therapy session and within the therapeutic relationship were operationalized, beginning with the particular *thematic content*. The second level comprised the clients' and therapists' *speech acts*, indicating a statement that a person directs to another person (Searle, 1969). The third level includes *episodes* consisting of different speech acts that contribute to client change and that can be clearly distinguished from all other therapeutic events. *Change events* are episodes that lead to subgoals (e.g., insight). If these change events can be repeatedly identified in one or more sessions, this then constitutes a change pattern. Greenberg (1986a) mentioned two different ways of identifying episodes or events. The first is a rational–empirical method, where, for example, the sessions of an experienced therapist are analyzed in order to identify change relevant events as in task analysis (Rice & Greenberg, 1984). The second method is purely empirical and consists of a sequential analysis of observational data to identify recurrent change events. We elaborate on these two methods in later sections of this chapter. Finally, the *relationship* level describes the qualities that the therapist and the client ascribe to their common interaction, and that can be extracted from the episodes and speech acts. We will limit ourselves to the level of the speech act and the relationship.

In the study of the strategies of social influence, themes that occur in an individual session have a secondary role. The central point of interest in the analysis is the speech acts. These acts can be classified, quantified and systematically observed, so it is possible to study the impact of specific types of speech acts on the behaviour or the experience of the other person. Of particular interest is the frequency of speech and how the episodes and speech acts contribute to therapeutic change.

In order to describe the interaction sequence on the level of speech acts or episodes, it is necessary to use systematic behavioural observation. However, the collection and analysis of observational data alone allows only for a description and analysis of the events at the behavioural level. If the impact of separate behavioural events is to be studied, then it is necessary to introduce a second-level dependent variable, that of the subjective experiences of both the therapist and client. Statements about helpful or unhelpful behavioural patterns can only be made if this pattern can be related in some meaningful way to the outcome of the session, of therapy, or to more specific sub-goals, such as compliance with homework assignments. According to this conceptual framework, process analysis encompasses both systematic behavioural observations as well as a systematic assessment of the experiences of the participants.

In this chapter we will expand further on the methodological aspects of a systematic assessment and outline those that are used to assess the different aspects of the therapeutic relationship.

Systematic observation of therapeutic interaction

Systematic observation can have many foci. The first focus is to describe what happens during a therapy session on the behavioural level. Secondly, through observation, it is possible to study the process of mutual influence in interaction and the mechanism of client behavioural change. Thirdly, researchers and trainees can relate behavioural patterns to success criteria (Hill, 1982). With these foci in mind, the level of the speech act seems appropriate for studying and describing behaviour (see also Herschbach, Klinger & Odefey, 1980). Accordingly, most observational studies choose this as the unit of investigation. However, a number of methodological points need to be considered. For example, in a speech act, three different aspects can be distinguished, i.e., the theme, the concrete action represented and the associated nonverbal qualities.

An important aspect of social influence is verbal interaction. Coding systems that enable researchers to study verbal interaction have received a great deal of attention in the literature. However, Kiesler (1982) emphasized that nonverbal communication is of greater importance and argued that verbal meanings vary according to their combination with different nonverbal signals. It is difficult to review systematically the different types of communication in all the reported studies, even when using simple codes such as a rating of positive, negative or neutral, because of the variety of different codes used in each study. It appears necessary, then, to study first the verbal aspects, since an exhaustive description of the total verbal and nonverbal therapeutic communication is not available. If change patterns that enable or hinder therapeutic progress are identified, then at a second stage, these could be studied in combination with different nonverbal signals.

In what follows, we will discuss the formal aspects of category formation and other methodological aspects of behavioural observation. Further, we describe the most important category systems and, finally, the methods of analysis.

Methodological aspects of behavioural observation

Formal aspects of category formation In developing category systems that can assess different speech acts, it is necessary to have an overriding formal taxonomic scheme that compares the different systems and provides for the construction of new ones (e.g., Rice, 1965; Rice & Wagstaff, 1967). Russell and Stiles (1979) have developed a classification that consists of three types of categories, namely content, intersubjective and extralinguistic; these may be distinguished using two coding strategies, classical and pragmatic.

Content categories relate to semantic or thematic content of words or groups of words. These constitute the first level in Greenberg's (1986a) conceptual framework, that of the thematic subject of a speech act. These categories produce a thematic representation of the therapy process. However, if one is interested in reciprocal interaction, these categories are inadequate. This is particularly so in psychoanalytically oriented studies where content categories have been distinguished.

Intersubjective categories describe the syntactic or otherwise implied relationship between sender and receiver. The category "Question", for example, implies that the person expects a certain class of information from the interaction partner and also implies that the person considers the situation to be one in which asking for this information is permissible. It is this intersubjective aspect of speech acts that offer the most useful information regarding the description and analysis of the therapeutic encounter; as a consequence, most category systems contain intersubjective categories.

The third category, *extralinguistic*, comprises nonverbal aspects of a speech act, such as laughing, stuttering or emphasis. Many category systems have been developed to measure these nonverbal communications as they are at least as important as, but also more often neglected than, the content and verbal categories.

For each of these three categories, a second criterion level of abstraction is introduced, consisting of the coding strategy that the observer uses when events have to be ordered into the categories. Following Berelson (1952) and Marsden (1965), it is possible to distinguish between the classical and pragmatic strategies.

In the *classical* strategy, the manifest content of a verbal statement is assessed. Berelson (1952) wished to limit content analysis to syntactic and semantic aspects of the utterance without inferences about it. In the classical model, objectivity is the prime criterion so as to enable the observer to carry out a content analysis with a minimum amount of training.

The *pragmatic* model addresses latent content, and focuses on the relationship between the person and their communication (Marsden, 1965), thus attempting to define the psychological significance of the communication. Since inferences are made on the level of coding, observers need more time to achieve acceptable levels of reliability. Whereas in the classical model, conclusions about the condition of the observed person can only be deduced after the process of coding and analyses, the pragmatic model allows for such inferences by the observer at the coding stage.

Both strategies have their advantages and disadvantages. The classical model does not require much observer training, but important aspects of the relationship can be neglected with the risk of arriving at conclusions that have little clinical relevance. The pragmatic strategy, in contrast, may be clinically relevant, but the researcher has to invest much in terms of training.

Every utterance can be ordered according to the two formal criteria, namely type of category and coding strategy. This classification is helpful in that it provides a summary of the coding systems most often used in the literature and is useful in the construction of new ones.

Defining the content of behavioural categories Though it is necessary to construct a system of behavioural categories, all observed behaviour must be divided into sequences of behavioural units that can be coded. In defining the categories, the system chosen or developed should satisfy a number of criteria. Systematic observation implies selection and abstraction. The choice of behavioural classes and their definitions should be derived from a theoretical model (Foster & Cone, 1986), so that the data can be used to test specific hypotheses.

Categories need to be constructed that describe those therapist and client behaviours that are assumed to be essential ingredients of influence or change, in order to be used for training counsellors and therapists. Goodman and

Table 6.1 Helping skills (Elliott et al, 1982a)

Category	Other name/subclass	Intention
Question	Open-closed information gathering	Gathering information
Advisement	Direct guidance: command, suggestion	Transferring guiding information
Reflection	Restatement, nonverbal referent	Communicating understanding message
Interpretation	Person—general exploration	Explaining help seeker to self
Self-disclosure	Me-too process	Deliberate sharing of self
Information	Edification, explanation	Explaining people who are not present or giving general information
Reassurance	Acknowledgement, confirmation	Supporting the help seeker and respond positively
Disagreement	Confrontation, criticism	Challenging or disagreeing
Silence/ interruption	Latency	Verbal allowing versus crowding

Dooley (1976) were the first to construct a system that described therapist behaviours. They arrived at a set of six separate categories which Elliot et al (1982a) increased to nine, based on more recent literature review. These behavioural classes are found in most category systems and are considered as essential helping skills. Table 6.1 provides a summary of these classes of therapist behaviour.

In addition to being derived from a theoretical model, categories should be exhaustive and independent. Exhaustiveness implies that all behaviours within the two-person interaction can be coded. For example, trends in mutual behavioural control can only be studied if the behaviour of both partners is included in a sequence. Most studies using systematic observation of therapeutic sessions have been limited to only therapist behaviour. Independence refers to categories being mutual, so that each behaviour can be unambiguously classified to one category only. The degree to which this criterion is satisfied, will determine largely the inter-observer reliability. Finally, the category should be described in behavioural terms and in a positive way, not as absence of behaviour.

Choice of the behavioural unit Having determined the behaviour categories, it is necessary to consider the unit of observation. Time sampling is not appropriate given that it fails to take into acount the continuity of therapist-client interaction. If the coding schemes are limited to just content categories, it is still necessary to choose the unit of observation.

These units vary from single words to utterances, to certain conversational themes. The unit most often described in the literature is the grammatical sentence, consisting of at least subject and predicate. Limitations such as these have their advantages, particularly regarding reliability, since agreement between observers is higher because of the more simple criteria. This is particularly the case when verbatim transcripts are coded. When coding is carried out directly from audio- or videotape, it is more difficult to identify grammatical sentences. A disadvantage of this unit of observation, is the fact that an utterance is artificially extracted and its meaning may thus change. Since the speaker's utterance often consists of more than one sentence, the alternating sequences of sender and receiver is lost, giving rise to considerable problems in the sequential analysis of the observational data.

Schaffer (1982) suggested that the coding unit should be defined as the contribution by client or therapist necessary to identify a "meaning unit". A new unit begins when, according to the definition of the category, the essence of the interaction changes, or when the interaction partner begins to speak. The choice of a meaning unit as unit of observation is preferable even if it requires more extensive observer training.

Choice of behavioural sample Process analysis studies are limited to the analysis of samples of one or more sessions. Sampling in this way poses two problems: *what* section of the session and *which* sessions should be sampled. Should sessions be selected after a certain point in time, for example after the second session, or after a certain theme, for example after discussing homework assignments? Since selection at a predetermined time in the sessions almost certainly result in a variation of themes, a sampling procedure using particular themes as criteria, seems the most preferable. Several studies have addressed the problem of generalizing from the results of studies with these samples. Kiesler, Matthieu and Klein (1965) showed that particular behaviours occur in different phases of a session, influenced mainly by the client's disturbance. Furthermore, they report only partial agreement between randomly selected samples and time-specific samples. Similar results were reported by Mintz and Luborsky (1971). In these studies global ratings were used rather than systematic observation.

Two points need to be considered here. Sessions can be segmented in different ways. So the conclusions drawn about the behaviour throughout the course of treatment will necessarily be tentative. Secondly, the choice of criteria used to select the most important sessions needs to be clear and be determined by the type of disturbance, as well as the programme. If one studies the predictive value of early sessions on outcome, then it may be appropriate to limit material just to these early sessions.

A review of existing category systems

Given that there is no common theoretical model of the process of change, each study has developed new categories according to different perspectives, making the comparison between studies problematic. This was highlighted in a systematic comparison of six coding systems (Elliott et al, 1987), in which seven therapy sessions were coded using a variety of different systems. Although the categories of each system could be ordered into the nine helping skills already mentioned, important differences in the ratings of these categories occurred. The authors found that even a similar label does not guarantee identical definitions and theoretical constructs, so that the comparison of results from studies using different coding schemes remains hazardous.

A complete analysis of the interaction and mutual control occurring between client and therapist requires the systematic observation of both client and therapist behaviour. A number of systems designed to code the client behaviour in therapy are available (Chamberlain, Patterson, Reid, Kavanagh, & Forgatch, 1984; Meier & Boivin, 1986). Only three of these systems, however, allow for the observation of both client and therapist behaviour (Hill, 1978;

Schindler, 1988; Stiles, 1978). Each is derived from a different theoretical perspective. The systems developed by Snyder (1945), Frank and Sweetland (1962), Stiles (1978) and Hochdörfer et al (1983) are based on client-centred therapy, while Hill (1978) and Schindler (1988) had a more eclectic approach, based on the psychotherapeutic process itself. In the one behaviourally oriented study, in which client behaviour was systematically observed (Chamberlain et al, 1984), only resisting behaviour was defined.

It is somewhat surprising that behaviour therapists, with a long and firm tradition in behavioural observation and in the development of observational instruments in other areas of research, have shown so little initiative in the application of behavioural observation to the process of psychotherapy. The only two exceptions are the studies by Ford (1978) on therapist behaviour and by Chamberlain et al (1984) on client behaviour.

Below we describe those category systems that have received most attention in the literature and that include intersubjective categories. We will summarize each coding system in terms of the methodological criteria outlined in the preceding sections of this chapter.

The Vanderbilt Psychotherapy Process Scale (VPPS) The VPPS was originally developed to obtain objective judgements about the characteristics and interaction of participants in the therapeutic process. The first version of the VPPS consisted of 84 Likert-type items that were scored on a five point ordinal scale. This version was used by Gomes-Schwartz and Schwartz (1978) to assess whether the instrument could discriminate between therapists from different schools. On the basis of an *a priori* content analysis, the items were divided into eight subscales that appeared internally consistent and that were highly reliable. Gomes-Schwartz (1978) later revised these into three factors, namely explorative processes, quality of the offered relationship and degree of client participation. Their original data were factor analysed yielding seven subscales that appeared to present a clear picture of the dimensions that were supposed to be predictors of outcome and that were internally consistent and reliable. This version consisted of 60 items and, in order to improve the reliability, a manual was constructed omitting items with low reliability and added some new items. These included three global ratings of the quality of the relationship, how productive the session seemed to be, and the client's present level of functioning (O'Malley, Suh & Strupp, 1983). The most recent version consists of 80 items and seven factors, six of which are identical to those in the first study: patient participation, patient hostility, therapist warmth, negative therapist attitude, patient exploration and therapist exploration. The seventh scale, patients' psychological distress, was mainly based on the items from the latest version. The internal consistency varied from alpha of 0.82 to 0.96, and the interrater agreement varied from 0.86 to 0.94.

The Penn Helping Alliance Counting Signs Method (HAcs) This method was developed for the Pennsylvania Psychotherapy Project to study the factors predictive of outcome. The HAcs is based on two important psychoanalytic concepts: the helping alliance and resistance. The HAcs consists of frequency counts from transcripts that are instances of certain forms of client expressions and that are indicative of a helping alliance. A manual was developed consisting of two general types of helping alliances, one where the client experiences the therapist as giving the necessary help, and one where the client experiences the treatment process with the therapist as cooperative and goal directed. Both types are divided into a number of positive and negative subtypes, constructed on the basis of pilot research and clinical literature (Luborsky, 1976). An independent observer determines all relevant client statements from a transcript, that is, signs that agree with the different subtypes of helping alliance. These are then classified and rated on a 5-point intensity scale. The score for each item is the sum of the signs in each session, weighted by the intensity rating. Three types of factors can be used: positive, negative and difference scores. The HAcs method was used on selected sessions from the 10 most and the 10 least successful of a total of 73 clients from the Penn Psychotherapy Project.

The Penn Helping Alliance Rating Method (HAR) was developed as a variation of the HAcs, in part due to the problems of reliability and validity. This instrument rates segments of sessions, and each item is rated on a 10-point Likert-type scale. The interrater reliability for the subscales varied from 0.75 to 0.88. The alpha coefficient, the coefficients for internal consistency, were 0.96 for the helping scales and 0.94 for the therapist-facilitating behaviour scales. The consistency of the HAR ratings of the early sessions with the later sessions were modest in general, but higher for the successful clients (0.69).

Structural Analysis of Social Behaviour (SASB) Benjamin (1974) presented a social behaviour psychological model that takes into account the description, explanation and prediction of social behaviour. The SASB model was developed to study social behaviours in different contexts. It consists of three different levels. The first addresses the relationship with another person and describes transitive behaviour that is directed towards another individual. The second level describes the relationship towards the self and contains an intransitive condition and reactions towards the behaviour of others. The third describes the individual's intrapsychic events. Each of these levels is superimposed on two further axes, affiliation and interdependence forming four quadrants, the points between the poles being the result of the relative influence of these two axes. From the way the SASB system is constructed, assumptions can be made about the complementarity and opposition within dyadic interactions. Benjamin (1982) described a cluster version of the SASB, in which the 36 points or behaviours from the first two levels comprise eight clusters.

The application of the SASB system in psychotherapy is illustrated in Benjamin (1979, 1982). Henry, Schacht and Strupp (1986) reported the use of the system in the comparison of one successful and one unsuccessful case from each of four therapists. The study is part of the Vanderbilt Psychotherapy Research Project (see Suh, Strupp & O'Malley, 1986) and on each occasion a 15-minute sample was used from the third session. The results indicated that the therapists in the successful cases showed more affirming/understanding and helping/protecting and less belittling/blaming. In the third session, succesful clients showed more disclosing/expressing, less trusting/relying and less walling off/avoiding.

Of all systems, the SASB best satisfies the requirement of theoretical derivation: yet this too is its main limitation. It is supposedly an instrument that analyses any social behaviour regardless of context. The categories reflect a high level of abstraction and therefore imply an extremely pragmatic coding strategy. From the results reported by Henry et al (1986) it is clear that the categories do not adequately fit the events that occur in the therapeutic process. The coding is extremely complex and time-consuming, so more convenient and economical systems tend to be used to study the process within therapeutic situations.

Verbal Response Modes (VRM) The VRM coding system has been developed to categorize communication in the context of client-centered psychotherapy. Goodman and Dooley (1976) identified six therapist response modes within psychotherapeutic interventions: *disclosure, question, silence, advisement, interpretation, reflection.* In using these six modes, the researchers encountered problems in distinguishing between advisement and interpretation. The first of three taxonomic principles was discovered when they realized that these categories could be discriminated on the basis of the answer to the following questions: Where does the idea discussed by the participants come from? Whose experience is described by the utterance?

An interpretation is related to the experience of the client or other, an advisement in contrast relates to the experience of the therapist. This taxonomic principle was then called "Source of Experience".

This principle seemed to distinguish the other categories as well. Advisement and disclosure are related to the experience of the therapist, whereas interpretation, question and reflection are related to the experience of the client. Silence poses problems, but we will return to this presently.

The second principle was discovered when the researchers tried to distinguish between reflection and interpretation. Both categories or modes referred to the client's experience but they are obviously quite different. The answer to the question "Whose frame of reference is referred to in the utterance?", seemed to discriminate between these two modes. Here again, the principle "Frame of reference", appeared to apply to the other modes as well.

Inspection of this scheme shows two immediate problems. First of all, there are empty cells which may indicate the existence of yet unknown categories and, secondly, each cell contains two different categories. In order that the therapist can offer a suggestion, an interpretation or a reflection, he/she has to have some knowledge about the client's experience. This produced the third principle, "Focus".

Two cells still remain empty. However, the missing categories can be construed on the basis of the three principles. If a cell concerns the therapist's experience, the client's frame of reference and is within the focus, then the client has to presume knowledge about the therapist's experience. If one assumes that this experience can be objective, then this category may contain objectively testable statements ("It is raining") and was called *edification* (statement of fact). The other empty cell concerns the therapist's experience, the frame of reference, with the focus on the client; the therapist has to assume knowledge about the client's experience. This category came to be known as *confirmation* and is coded in utterances such as "We do not agree with each other", which might be translated as: "I am not talking about my own ideas, but I assume that I know yours". This leaves the problem of *silence*. Originally, this category contained both pauses and nonlexical utterances. These vocalized pauses indicate that one is listening: this category was then called acknowledgment. Finally, it became clear that this taxonomy could be used in any type of discourse so the names client and therapist were changed into other and speaker.

Thus far the VRM is described as a system that categorizes the interpersonal intent of utterances. However, each utterance also has a specific grammatical form. For example, "Would you close the door?" could be coded on intent level as advisement; the grammatical form, however, is a question which is more polite than a direct request or a demand. Table 6.2 gives a summary of the grammatical form, as described within the VRM system.

Table 6.2   The Verbal Response Modes (Form)

Disclosure	Declarative; first person singular
Question	Interrogative; inverted subject–verb order
Edification	Declarative; third person
Acknowledgement	Nonlexical; contentless terms of address
Advisement	Imperative; verbs of permission, obligation
Interpretation	Second person; implication of an attribute
Confirmation	First person plural; listener is included
Reflection	Second person; implication of internal experience or cognitive action

In addition to quantifying discourse in terms of the different categories, the VRM system is able to describe and categorize any social encounter in yet another way. It is possible to calculate the proportion of the utterance pertaining to (1) the experience of the speaker, (2) the other, (3) the speaker's frame of reference, (4) the other, (5) the speaker's focus, (6) the other. These categories expressed in terms of the three taxonomic principles are referred to as *role dimensions*, which form the poles of three bipolar dimensions that can b   e distinguished on the intent level. They are referred to as informativeness/ attentiveness, presumptuousness/non-presumptuousness, and acquiesence/ directiveness.

The VRM coding system has thus far been used in a number of studies (Schaap & Suntjes, 1986; Stiles, 1979; Stiles & Sultan, 1979; Stiles, McDaniel & McGaughey, 1979), all of which investigated the differences between contrasting therapeutical orientations. This system is not without its limitations: although the categories are derived and defined on the basis of formal theoretical principles, they are heterogeneous with regard to content. The disclosure category for example, contains such diverse features as feelings, wishes and opinions. The interpretation category is a combination of self-disclosure, feedback, interpretation and trust, as exemplified in the manual (Stiles, 1978). The coding system contains 64 categories (any combination of eight categories on intent and eight on form level), which is too many for both frequency and sequential analysis.

The category system of Elliott (1979) This system is comprised of categories that only code therapist behaviour and is based on the helping skills literature. It contains only intersubjective categories, with the exception of questions implying a pragmatic coding strategy. The unit of observation is defined grammatically as a complete sentence (Table 6.3).

In the three studies in which the system has been used, the categories are not mutually exclusive (Elliott et al, 1982a). Elliott based this procedure on

Table 6.3   The category system for therapist behaviour (based on Elliott, 1979)

Closed Question
Open Question
General advisement
Process advisement
Reflection
Interpretation
Reassurance
Disagreement
Self-disclosure
Information

Labov and Fanshel (1977) who argued that one statement may contain more than one of the 10 categories; therefore each unit of observation is rated on a 4-point rating scale (from 0 = clearly absent to 3 = clearly present) on each of the 10 categories or dimensions. The inter-observer agreement can only be calculated using a correlation between observers per dimension and this correlation varies between 0.77 and 0.91. The studies listed were on the impact of particular therapist behaviour on the client's experience.

Shapiro, Barkham and Irving (1984) have slightly modified the system by introducing an exploration category. They treat the categories as mutually exclusive and report an overall kappa reliability coefficient for 12 sessions of 0.76.

In contrast to the other systems, this one was specifically developed to be of use in therapeutic situations. The categories are based on assumptions about helping skills or necessary therapeutic skills. The system does not include client behaviour because the focus is on the client's experience and concrete therapist behaviours that lead to positive client experience.

The disadvantage of the system lies in the multiple rating of each behavioural unit, yielding a combination of observation and ratings, which complicates the interpretation of the results.

The Counselor and Client Verbal Response Coding System (CCVRCS)
This system developed by Hill (Hill et al, 1981) contains subsystems for both therapist and client behaviour. The categories have not been derived from a theoretical perspective but are common to most coding systems. The final category system, described in the manual, was constructed in a number of steps on the basis of trial coding.

Hill started by comparing the categories and definitions of 11 existing coding systems and produced a list of 25 separate categories. For each of these, a definition was written out with examples taken from the original coding manuals. Two raters used this version in coding two sessions yielding a low inter-observer reliability. In a second version, the least reliable categories were omitted and a new category nonverbal Referent was included, but this did not increase reliability. In the third version, the definitions were improved, the examples were expanded, and a new category was added, that of Aside, (explanation by procedures). This version produced improved and satisfactory levels of reliability and, in order to test the validity of the system, the categories were presented to three raters with a list of examples of all categories in a random order. They were instructed to order each example in the correct category. In only half of the examples, were two out of the three raters able to do so correctly, indicating that the definitions lacked clarity. This led to a fourth version, in which the categories with the least agreement were omitted. The validity of this version, containing 17 categories, was tested using the same procedure. In 80% of the cases, two out of three raters were able to order the examples within the correct definitions. An analysis of the discrepancies resulted in a fifth version, in which the definitions of the 17 categories were adopted. In the sixth phase of development of the system, 12 intake sessions were analysed and on the basis of a cluster analysis, the 17 categories were reduced to 14, summarized in five dimensions.

The client behaviour subsystem consists of nine categories, on the basis of the coding system developed by Snyder (1945). The development of the category definitions and examples is much less extensively described than that of the therapist subsystem. The process was similar to that described above and took place in four steps. The categories are presented in Table 6.4.

In this system it is necessary to transcribe the conversation verbatim. The unit of behaviour used is the grammatical sentence and a period of 20 hours is required for training the observers. Hill (1978) studied the reliability of the validity of the therapist behaviours. Twelve intakes were coded, with the kappa coefficient of reliability varying between 0.79 and 0.81.

Based on the criteria described above, this can be described as the best available system. The heterogeneity of the categories is less of a problem since they are all relevant to therapeutic situations. The categories coding client behaviour

Table 6.4   The Client and Therapist Verbal Response Coding System (based on Hill et al, 1981)

Therapist categories	Client categories
Minimal responses	*Simple responses*
Minimal Encourager	Requests
Silence	Descriptions
Directives	*Experiencing*
Approval–Reassurance	Exploration of counsellor–client
Information	relationship
Direct guidance	*Insight*
Questions	Discussions of plans
Closed Questions	*Silence*
Open Questions	Other
Complex reactions	
Restatement	
Reflection	
Interpretation	
Confrontation	
Strange bedfellows	
Nonverbal Referent	
Self-disclosure	
Other	

are less detailed than those for therapist behaviour, nevertheless the system does provide a more complete account of therapeutic interactions and permit sequential analysis (Hill et al, 1983).

The Coding System of Interaction in Psychotherapy (CIP) The CIP was constructed with the aim of fulfilling the conditions of a theoretical deduction and sequential analysis. The category system is on the level of verbal responses. The choice of categories was determined partly by assumptions about client and therapist behaviour (e.g., Kanfer & Grimm, 1980; Kanfer & Schefft, 1988) and partly by existing category systems, to make comparisons between different psychotherapeutic schools possible. According to the criteria presented by Russell and Stiles (1979), the categories of the CIP are to be rated as intersubjective. Some categories, however, also include thematic content, e.g., Feelings and Message of Success. As is the case with the preceding coding system of Hill

Table 6.5   The Coding System for Interaction in Psychotherapy (based on Schindler et al, 1988)

Therapist categories	Client categories
Empathy	*Self-disclosure*
Feeling reflection	Description of positive feeling
Reformulation	
Understanding	Description of negative feeling
Support	Proposal
Minimal support	*Trust*
Encouragement	*Problem description*
Positive feedback	Factual message
Exploration	*Specific description*
Asking for information	Simple responses
Summarizing	Short response
Factual message	Own activity
Directivity	Asking for advice
Structuring	*Plan for change*
Explaining	Self-control attempt
Assignment in therapy	Message of success
Assignment outside therapy	Insight
Classified attitude	Therapeutic relationship
Confrontation	*Inhibiting behaviour*
Interpretation	Refusal–avoidance
Criticism	Criticism–provocation
Self-disclosure	Resignation
Other	*Other*
Listening	Listening
Pause	Pause
Rest	*Rest*

et al (1981), the coding strategy falls between the so-called classical and pragmatic approach (Marsden, 1965), since a category is not only defined by grammatical criteria but often by an intention or its context as well.

The CIP contains two different subsystems, one for the therapist and one for the client behaviour. A short description of the categories is included in Table 6.5. For a comprehensive description of the categories, see Schindler, Hohenberger-Sieber and Hahlweg (1989).

The subsystem of therapist behaviour contains a total of 20 categories and is based to a large extent on the systems decribed by Suh, Strupp & O'Malley (1986) and Hill et al (1981). The client subsystem contains a total of 19 categories and is based to a large extent on the observation systems of Snyder (1945), Hahlweg et al (1984), and Hill et al (1981). The observational unit was defined as the act within the total utterance of the person.

The CIP is a differentiated system. The relatively high number of categories, however, gives it the disadvantage that the frequency of single categories may be very low indeed. A solution to this problem consists of combining similar categories into a super-category. This is made possible by the dimensions that are distinguished within the category system.

The first form reduces the super-categories into three comprehensive categories each time. For the therapist this consists of a category combining the gathering and giving of information (Exploration/Explanation), a combination of Empathy and Support, and Directivity and Classification. For the client Short Answer and Problem Description were combined. The second comprehensive category consists of all behaviours that have to do with Initiative, Cooperation and constructive contributions of the client. The third category Inhibiting Behaviour remains a separate category.

The second form of reduction (II) was necessary to be able to depict the course of interaction within one session in a point graph (Gottman, 1979; Schaap, 1982). In order to construct point graphs, categories have to be reduced to positive, neutral and negative behaviours.

The reliability and validity of the CIP was then studied in a sample of 64 intake sessions (Schindler et al, 1989). Reliability was high for both therapist categories (kappa = 0.80) and client categories (kappa = 0.79). The course of these structured interviews could be decribed successfully with the categories of the CIP. Evidence for the validity of the CIP was provided by the correlations between subjective ratings of clients and therapists and the different behavioural categories. For instance, between the therapist rating of the client's self-disclosure and the client's actual Feeling Utterances as coded by the CIP.

The CIP was then studied in a number of process studies where complete therapies were analysed. Kaimer, Reinecker and Schindler (1989) studied also a successful and unsuccessful case treated by the same therapist. The change in behaviour during the course of treatment could be described, as well as other systematic effects in the conversational feedback system. These results could be replicated and were expanded in a comprehensive process study with 34 complete therapies (Schindler, 1988, 1990).

Sequential analysis of observational data

Most studies on client-therapist interaction using behavioural observation, have used methods of analysis that are limited to frequencies of certain behavioural classes. Usually, sections from particular sessions are sampled, coded and then correlated with different process variables. Although these frequency analyses are important, they are somewhat limited in describing changes in the client and therapist behavioural pattern during a session or over a series of sessions. The study of category frequencies therefore does not describe the regularities or laws that may govern the mutual control that exists between the client and therapist conversations. Tracking how particular therapist behaviours influence subsequent client behaviour is necessary and has led to innovative methodological procedures (see Elliott, 1983; Fiske, 1977; Kiesler, 1979; Zimmer, 1983).

Snyder (1945) was the first to study the direct impact of therapist behaviour. Several studies have been reported since using comparable methodological analyses and a few have reported on client-therapist first-order transition probabilities (see Russell & Trull, 1986). However, there are no studies in which the interaction pattern over longer sequences has been analysed, an analytic procedure that has been used successfully for almost a decade in marital and family communication research (Gottman, 1979; Hahlweg, Revenstorf & Schindler, 1984; Patterson, 1982; Schaap, 1982). In order to use this method of analysis, the data have to be collected in a particular way.

In order to study how the clients and therapists mutually control each others' behaviours and interaction, it is necessary to code client and therapist behaviours and maintain the speaker–listener sequences. If the grammatical sentence is chosen as the unit of observation, then a sequence of categories for each person usually emerges, but what remains problematic, is the identification of the stimulus or antecedent behaviour for which the response of the other is the consequent event. The category system should therefore order a unit of behaviour unambiguously into one class of behaviour.

The first step in sequential analysis is to calculate the immediate contingencies between two classes of behaviour. These contingencies are the first-order transitions and describe the probability that the client will respond contingently with a particular class of behaviour e.g., self-disclosure, in response to a given stimulus event, say therapist empathy. A contingency between these two classes of behaviour is established if the conditional probability (e.g., empathy) for self-disclosure is greater than its unconditional probability or base rate. The differences between the conditional probability and the base rate of the consequent behaviour can be statistically tested (Margolin and Wampold, 1981; Revenstorf, Hahlweg, Schindler & Vogel, 1984; Sackett, 1978; see also Allison & Liker, 1982).

These immediate contingencies between one behavioural class and the consequent behaviour present events of relatively short duration. Interaction patterns over longer periods of time and with more utterances are usually more interesting and describe the level of episodes (Greenberg, 1986a).

For such an analysis of these sequences, two approaches have been developed, Lag Sequential Analysis (LSA; Sackett, 1978) and N-Gram Analysis (NGA; Revenstorf et al, 1984). A critical comparison of both approaches is offered in Henrich and Hahlweg (1987).

Instruments measuring the subjective experience of the therapeutic relationship

The various methodologies described above enable researchers to investigate various aspects of verbal behaviour within therapeutic interventions. However, as therapeutic change becomes evident, it is important to know what subjective experience is correlated with successful change and what interaction patterns are associated with these experiences.

Greenberg (1986a) distinguishes between three levels of abstraction with regard to therapeutic success: the immediate impact of particular therapist behaviours; the indirect effect; and the outcome at the end of treatment.

On the level of subjective experience, the immediate impact of therapist behaviour consists of the experience of that behaviour or relevant episodes. The indirect effect is related to the experience of a whole session and the outcome is assessed using appropriate methods. The following instruments enable researchers or therapists to assess the subjective aspects within therapeutic encounters.

The experience of particular behaviours

Interpersonal Process Recall (IPR) It is impossible to assess directly the way a particular therapist behaviour affects the client without interfering with the course of the therapeutic conversation. It is possible however to record the session and use the tape as a stimulus to recall the impact of particular behaviours or episodes. This method of Interpersonal Process Recall was developed by Kagan, Krathwohl and Miller (1963) as a procedure to train counsellors. It provides unstructured feedback but can be used in a more systematic way to analyse client-therapist interaction (see for instance Elliott, 1984, 1986).

Immediately after the session, the therapist and client separately watch the recorded interaction in the presence of the researcher. Segments or whole sessions are shown and the client is instructed to rate each therapist behaviour in terms of his/her subjective experience. Different aspects of the therapeutic relationship have been studied in this way. Elliott (1979) instructed clients to indicate the intention behind particular therapist behaviours, then these were ordered on the basis of content criteria into one of six intention categories (see also Stiles, 1986; Elliott et al, 1982b; Fuller & Hill, 1985).

The IPR is an interesting method since it enables participants to assess the subjective experience of particular behaviour, but it does rely on the client's capacity to remember the impact of particular events without a session. A similar procedure was used by Schaap (1982) in the context of marital interaction (see also Schaap, 1984; Schaap & Jansen-Nawas, 1985; Schaap, Buunk & Kerkstra, 1988).

The experience of a whole session

Process and outcome research should ideally describe and analyse the course of therapy from a session, as well as relate the outcome of individual sessions to the overall outcome (Greenberg, 1986b). Studies requiring client-therapist and independent observers to rate qualities of a session, have reported modest agreement (e.g., Mintz, Auerbach, Luborsky & Johnson, 1973). The instruments following were developed for participants to judge the quality of their interaction.

Therapy Session Report (TSR) Orlinsky and Howard (1966) developed the TSR to assess many different aspects of the client's and therapist's experience. They were interested in the whole spectrum of the experience and included the following areas in the (client) form:

- the total rating of the session,
- a survey of themes covered,
- expected outcome of the session,
- own behaviour during the session,
- own feelings during the session,
- qualitative development during the session,

- satisfaction during the session,
- therapist behaviour during the session,
- therapist feelings during the session.

As is reflected in the choice of the items, the instrument is psychoanalytically oriented, with both the content-related items and relationship issues based on psychoanalytic constructs. Orlinsky and Howard (1975) presented a summary of the factorial structure of the TSR, as well as the correlations between the factors with the criterion and group comparisons. The sample consisted of 60 patients and 17 therapists who rated several sessions using the TSR. The aim was to reaching an exhaustive description of the experience of a session and the factor analysis was set to extract the maximal number of significant factors. The analysis produced 45 factors for the client version and 43 for the therapist version. The factors reflect the contribution of both participants, rather than assess the impression or the outcome of the session.

Session Evaluation Questionnaire (SEQ) Whereas Orlinsky and Howard (1975) attempted to describe the experience of the therapy session as extensively as possible, Stiles (1980) developed the SEQ so that the session could be considered as the unit of experience. The SEQ consists of two parts, one giving a rating of the session and the other rating the feelings associated with it. Both parts contain 11 pairs of adjectives and, in the construction, care was taken to include the three classical factors of the Semantic Differential, namely the evaluation, potency, and activity (Osgood, May & Miron, 1975) as well as different emotions.

A total of 16 therapists gave the SEQ to their clients at the end of one or more sessions and also rated these sessions themselves. The total sample consisted of 113 sessions, rated by both client and therapist. The clients' and therapists' scores were factor analysed separately; the first questionnaire (Rating of the session) produced two independent factors—Depth/Value and Smoothness/Ease—with this factor structure being almost identical for the client and therapist responses.

The second part of the questionnaire (Feelings associated with the session) resulted in one factor, Positive Feelings. This was positively and significantly correlated with both factors from the first part for both clients and therapists. A different relationship was reported for positive feelings between clients and therapists. Therapists felt better after sessions that clients rated as deep and useful, whereas clients felt better after sessions that the therapist rated as frictionless and easy. Similar discrepancies were reported by Orlinsky and Howard (1975), who concluded that the ways therapists experience the relationship was an inappropriate indicator of the clients' experience.

In another study, the stability of the factors over several sessions was tested (Stiles & Snow, 1984). Using 17 therapists, a total sample of 942 sessions were rated after adding two items to the questionnaire. The first part of the questionnaire yielded the same factor structure whereas analyses of the second part yielded two factors, positive feelings and arousal. Comparisons between sessions indicated that the factor structure remained stable.

Fuller and Hill (1985) used both factors from the first part of the SEQ to test the relationship between the experience of the session and process characteristics. Here again differences between clients and therapists were reported. Clients rated a session as agreeable and frictionless when they recognised the therapist's supportive intentions, whereas therapists rated sessions in this way if problem solving went smoothly. This study showed that therapists and clients give different meanings to individual process characteristics.

The experience of the person

The quality of the therapeutic relationship can be operationalized from both partners' contribution. In the same way that outcome can be rated, behavioural style also has perspectives that can be distinguished: the perceptions of the client, the therapist and of an independent observer.

Most studies have used the independent observer ratings (for an overview, see Alexander & Luborsky, 1986; Gurman, 1977; Suh et al, 1986) and have shown that the quality of a therapeutic relationship has an important impact on outcome. Those studies where ratings of therapists, client and observer were compared report little interrater agreement (Gurman, 1977), suggesting that, on each occasion that the relationship was rated, different characteristics were of importance depending on the person's perspective.

Truax and Carkhuff (1967) argued that the clients are incapable of perceiving the relevant nuances in the therapeutic relationship because of their particular presenting problems. This position inevitably leads to an over-reliance on independent observers' ratings, even though several studies have shown that the interpersonal perception of both client and therapist is important in defining the course and outcome of treatment (Ford, 1978; Hoogduin et al, 1988; Rabavilas et al, 1979; Saltzman, Luetgert, Roth & Howard, 1976).

The following instruments were developed to assess the participants' interpersonal perception of the therapy process.

The Lorr scales   These scales were developed to assess the feelings and attitudes that clients have about their therapists (Lorr, 1965). It was assumed that the way the clients perceived their therapist is a good predictor of the way they behave. Based on the ideas of Fiedler (1950) and Leary (1957), an inventory was constructed with eight perceptual dimensions rated on 65 items. The items were formulated to describe the client's experience ("He understands me, even though I do not express myself clearly"). The original items were presented to a sample of 523 patients producing five factors: Understanding, Accepting, Authoritarian, Independence-encouraging, and Critical–Hostile.

Lorr (1965) reported correlations between these factors and client change. Understanding and Accepting correlated most positively with ratings of change, whereas Authoritarian and Critical–Hostile negatively correlated. Sloane et al (1975) used this scale in their study comparing behaviour therapy and psychoanalytic psychotherapy and found no differences between the two approaches in the client's rating at the end of therapy.

Relationship Inventory (RI) This instrument was developed by Barrett-Lennard (1986), enabling clients to rate their therapists. Although in most studies clients rate their therapists, therapists too have also been asked to rate their clients. The inventory was developed utilizing Rogerian principles assuming that the essential effective ingredient of therapist behaviour is the way they are perceived by the clients. The inventory has four subscales: Empathy, Congruence, Level of Regard, and Unconditional Regard.

Gurman (1977) reviewed 14 studies using the RI and reported average internal consistencies varying from 0.74 to 0.81 for the various subscales. The 10 studies reporting test-retest reliability also showed a high degree of stability with average correlations for the different subscales varying from 0.80 to 0.90. Gurman concluded that although the different subscales show some overlap, they do measure consistently different dimensions of the perception of the therapeutic relationship. Factor analytic studies on the basis of item-intercorrelations also suggest that the RI does indeed assess different dimensions that are consistent with the original work by Barret-Lennard.

Therapeutic Alliance Scales (TAS) Marziali, Marmar and Krupnick (1981) developed an instrument that could be used by independent judges in rating therapeutic relationships. It was later extended to assess both clients' and therapists' subjective experience. Although the items for the client, therapist and observer have the same content, each formulation is somewhat different. Marziali (1984) reported on 42 cases using the scale which was completed after every session and on several occasions during therapy. The scales were presented each time after the session had ended, and several times for each therapy. In contrast to the results from other studies, there was relative agreement in the ratings of the client, therapist and observer, with a positive correlation between the quality of the therapeutic relationship and treatment outcome.

The Impact Message Inventory (IMI) The IMI gives a profile of the existing affective, cognitive and behavioural relationship of one person towards another. The main assumption behind the construction of the inventory was that the relationship is inevitable and pervasive in human interaction and is mainly established through the nonverbal messages that people send to one another. The central constructs are the evoking message (Beier, 1966) and the impact message (Kiesler, 1982). The *evoking message* is a condition or request which determines how the receiver of the message behaves, whereas the *impact message* determines how messages are received. The latter therefore reflects the subtle affective, cognitive and behavioural influences that are generated by the recipient as a result of the evoking message. The IMI is based on the assumption that the person's interpersonal style can be measured reliably by determining the covert responses evoked by his/her interaction partner.

The first version of the IMI of 259 items was based on the Interpersonal Behaviour Inventory (Lorr & McNair, 1965). The number of items for each of the 15 interpersonal styles varied from 12 to 21 and, for each item, a 4-point scale was constructed. First use of this instrument produced a later version consisting of 82 items and these were divided into three subclasses of impacts messages: Direct Feelings, Action Tendencies and Perceived Evoking Message. The internal consistency of each of the 15 subscales was studied by correlating the item score with the average score for the subscale, which yielded high correlation coefficients (Perkins et al, 1979). After a further factor analysis, three factors were identified that together explained 85% of the total variance, these being dominance or status, affiliation, and submissiveness. Research indicated that the 15 interpersonal subscales could be ordered in a circumplex model (Perkins et al, 1979).

Therapist and Client Rating Scale (TCRS) Schindler et al (1983), in the context of the Munich Marital Therapy Study (Hahlweg & Jacobson, 1984), developed a first version of a Therapist Rating Scale. This scale enabled clients to indicate their personal impression about the behaviour of their therapist on 27 bipolar items. The items were devised on the basis of two dimensions: Empathy/Understanding and Directivity/Structuring. The 10-point items were rated by a total of 200 subjects at the end of marital therapy by a total of seven therapists. Factor analysis yielded three factors: Empathy, Directivity and Activity. Results indicated moreover that clients who participated successfully in a reciprocity training rated their therapists higher in all three scales than those with negative results.

Since the internal consistency of all three factors in this first version was relatively low, the rating scale was improved in an effort to find more homogeneous factors (Hahlweg, Langlotz & Schindler, 1983). The scale was expanded to 41 items and completed by 115 patients of a psychosomatic clinic after therapy. A parallel form was completed by their therapists. A total of 16 therapists participated in this study. The outcome criteria consisted of success ratings by client and therapist, as well as an instrument developed and described in Zielke and Kopf-Mehnert (1978).

Factor analysis of the ratings by the clients yielded the following three factors with a high internal consistency: Sympathy/Interest (alpha = 0.91), Competence (alpha = 0.84) and Directivity (alpha = 0.89). Factor analysis of the ratings by the therapists also yielded three factors with a different selection and combination of items though: Sympathy (alpha = 0.92), Self-disclosure (alpha = 0.87) and Co-operation/Target-orientation (alpha = 0.89). All factors showed a high internal consistency. Moreover, significant correlations were found between the therapist and client factors, on the one hand, and outcome, based on client ratings, on the other hand. Similar correlations were found with outcome from the perspective of the therapist.

In the context of a transcultural study, these scales were translated into English. A total of 49 clients in a counselling setting in England completed the form. Factors showed a comparable internal consistency and significant correlations with the success criteria (Bennun, Hahlweg, Schindler & Langlotz, 1986). The therapist and client factors yielded moreover high correlations (average $r = 0.87$).

The positive correlations with outcome should be interpreted somewhat carefully since outcome was rated at the end of treatment together with the rating of the person of the therapist or client. A similar relationship would be shown if the rating of the person took place in an earlier phase of treatment.

This was the case in a study reported by Bennun and Schindler (1988) of a homogeneous group of 35 phobic patients treated by five therapists over an average of 10 sessions. After the second session both client and therapist completed the rating scale. The outcome criterion was the score on the Fear Survey Schedule and a judgement of both therapist and client about success of treatment. Significant correlations were reported between outcome and the three client and therapist factors. Although this study seems to suggest that the mutual rating of client and therapist in an early phase of treatment is related to outcome, a number of studies in different centres in the Netherlands question the validity of this statement. In a study comparing the predictive power of the subscales Empathy (E), Positive Regard (P), Incongruency (I), and Negative Regard (N), referred to as EPIN, of the Relationship Inventory (Lietaer, 1976), and the TCRS (Keijsers, Schaap, Hoogduin & Peters, 1991) for 36 patients with anxiety disorders, only the client assessment of the quality of the therapeutic relationship by EPIN was found to be related to treatment outcome. Neither the EPIN therapist form nor the TCRS showed a significant correlation. Therefore, the value of the TCRS still has to be demonstrated in further research, the more so since Keijsers, Schaap and Hoogduin (1992), in a study on 51 outpatients, reported serious methodological problems and a factor structure different from the

German and British studies.

Considerations in designing process outcome research

The preceding paragraphs of this chapter contain considerations of the process variables that should be studied, the degree of complexity of the data analysis, and methods for yielding and analysing sequential data. Connected with this is the question about the ideal research strategy. Zimmer (1983) classifies the studies reported in the literature into the following different experimental designs.

Analogue studies

This form is appropriate for testing the effect of individual behavioural patterns (e.g., Kanfer et al, 1960; Mann & Murphy, 1975). A standardization of the situation is possible, as well as an optimal experimental variation of the variables studied. Because of the isolation of individual variables, this is however effectuated at the cost of a loss of relevance in the clinical situation and, consequently, in transfer to the practical therapeutic situation. Results from analogue studies should therefore be replicated in clinical studies. A further limitation lies in the fact that analogue studies usually only apply to the initial phase of treatment. Later phases of treatment are almost impossible to simulate since the relevant context is difficult to manage.

Post hoc analyses

In this type of study, therapist and client both judge each other at the end of treatment. Examples are provided by Bennun et al (1986), Blanchard et al (1983), Rabavilas et al (1979), Hoogduin, de Haan and Schaap (1989). These ratings are then related to outcome measurements. Such retrospective ratings constitute surely a very global index for the therapeutic relationship and its impact on the course of treatment. Only rough styles of behaviour are derived in this way and no conclusions can be drawn about changes in the course of treatment. The rating of the relationship, no doubt strongly influenced by the positive or negative result of treatment, will probably reflect momentary experiences.

Systematic variation of therapist behaviour

Although these studies impress by their experimental nature, a number of disadvantages can be pointed out. Usually therapeutic style, such as Warmth–Coldness (Morris & Suckermann, 1974) or Authoritarian–Democratic (Ringler, 1977) is varied. In the case that one therapist should use both styles, one could rightly question his or her ability to do so. Furthermore, some ethical issues have been circumvented by using nonclinical samples, thereby causing the same problems in generalizations as have already been pointed out for analogue research.

Naturalistic comparative studies

In these studies several therapists or methods of treatment are compared without keeping constant essential variables such as duration and content. Examples are Sloane et al (1975) and Arentewicz and Schmidt (1980). The significance of the therapeutic relationship is difficult to prove in these studies: its impact is hard to judge because the variables are not kept constant. However, it would be possible in the long run after a large number of clients have been treated by the same therapist, to select successful cases and failures and compare these on the basis of process features.

Process outcome studies with different levels of measurement

This form of research enables the study of concrete behaviour during the sessions in the course of treatment. Comparable patients are treated within the same treatment program. The actual behaviour in the session is analysed, as well as the personal experience of the session by client and therapist (e.g., Ford, 1978). By measuring reliably and validly outcome at the same time, outcome can be related to specific process parameters. The study reported in Hill et al (1988) is an example of this intensive research strategy, even if the therapy with regard to duration and content was not equal for the eight patients included.

Implications

To be able to indicate the type of intervention, i.e., the specific therapist behaviour, for a specific problem with a specific client, much empirical data must still be gathered. According to our (short) review of research strategies, analogue studies and studies experimentally varying behaviour style will furnish information about strategies of social influence. However, as is the case with naturalistic comparative studies, these studies will be limited and must be considered as contributing in a minor way to process–outcome studies. No doubt, this last research strategy, also the most intensive one, will yield the most valuable results. Ideally the following criteria should be used to set up such a study.

1   A homogeneous group of patients should be studied. One must assume that different diagnostic categories will to a differing extent evoke treatment strategies at different times.
2   The therapists should have a comparable level of training. Also, the treatment should be kept constant with regard to content and duration. Only when the intervention techniques are standardized can the impact of social interaction reliably be studied.
3   The first level of measurement is the concrete behaviour of client and therapist during the session. This should be objectively measured and quantitatively processed. To be able to do so, a behavioural–observational method should be used that enables the description of the process of interaction. Since the first target should consist of the description of behavioural patterns and changes over time, a complete and continuous registration of one session as well as the whole course of treatment is necessary. Only on the basis of such data will it be possible to assess the significance of different phases. Later research could then be limited to such phases. Such a data gathering technique makes sequential analysis possible and, consequently, the study of mutual influence in interaction.
4   A category system to code therapeutic interaction should be used that enables the recording of the behaviour of both interaction partners, distinguishes between the therapist behaviour classes that are emphasized in behavioural psychotherapy and makes sequential analysis possible. Such information on a behavioural level is the prerequisite for the often woeful lack of more complex events (e.g., Cousins & Power, 1986; Greenberg, 1986a).
5   The second level of measurement consists of the subjective experience of client and therapist. Of interest is the association between the experience of the other person during a session and therapeutic outcome. Further, the data on both levels of measurement can be related, for instance yielding the behavioural correlates of constructive or destructive experiences during sessions. Once all these conditions been fulfilled then the outcome of treatment has to be assessed adequately in order to relate this to the process parameters and experiences of sessions.

These conditions represent the ideal process–outcome study. No study thus far encountered in the literature fulfils all of these conditions adequately. This considerably limits the power of the propositions one could base on these studies. Nevertheless, in the next chapter, we will attempt to review the available literature on different aspects of the therapeutic relationship.

7 Empirical findings on the level of verbal interaction

Introduction

The previous chapter described different methods and instruments used to study psychotherapy and the therapeutic relationship. This chapter will focus on the findings of studies that have used these procedures. More specifically, research will be presented that examines the relationship between behavioural style and treatment outcome, and on studies using behavioural observational measures.

Global ratings of behavioural style

Client behavioural characteristics

Goldfried (1982) presented a description of client behavioural characteristics that are considered to be conditions for a successful course of therapy. Some of these include:

1 The belief that change is possible and that it occurs slowly and in small steps (*expectancy*).
2 Accepting responsibility and participating actively in therapy (*motivation*).
3 Being prepared to discuss problems openly during the session (*self-exploration*).
4 Agreement to participate in exercises (e.g., role play) and accept the necessary feedback (*openness*).
5 Following therapeutic assignments between sessions (*transfer/generalization*).

The construct of *expectancy* emerged from literature on the placebo effect (Rosenthal & Frank, 1956). A distinction must be made between expectancies about outcome and expectancies about the process of therapy (Goldstein, 1962). With regard to outcome expectancies, a number of studies have been conducted in the area of systematic desensitization. It is important to note two different aspects of expectancies (Wilkins, 1973): that is, expectancy can be considered a stable characteristic that the client brings into treatment and which in part determines outcome; alternatively, it can be induced through therapist instructions and therefore can be considered as an independent variable. The difference in therapeutic success between the two groups (high versus low expectancy) can be linked to expectancy as a mediating variable, but usually the differences found in therapeutic success have not been significant (Wilkins, 1973).

The influence of initial expectancy of success on actual outcome has not been sufficiently demonstrated (see also Kazdin & Wilcoxon, 1976; Lick & Bootzin, 1975; Wilkins, 1973). Wilkins (1973) questioned whether expectancy needs further study on a behavioural level, i.e. whether an observable pattern can be identified that co-determines therapeutic change. What remains important is the way that therapists induce positive expectancies and facilitate a good outcome.

Client expectancies may also be important when considering role behaviour in therapy. A number of studies have investigated the extent to which disappointment has an adverse effect on treatment outcome. In their survey, Duckro, Beal and George (1979) noted that most studies failed to specify if expectancy referred to what the client ideally wished or what was anticipated. It is therefore not surprising that in about half of the studies, a positive relationship was found between disappointing expectancies and negative consequences for outcome. Benbenishty (1987) found that the discrepancy between expectancy and actual therapist behaviour decreased from the first session to later sessions. No analyses have been reported on in regard to outcome but, overall, studies show that, in successful treatment, changes in expectancy occur during the first few sessions, which may indicate that it simply becomes more realistic.

The construct of *motivation* is similar to expectancy, in that the same type of methodological problems are encountered in research. Motivation for psychotherapy is defined in a number of ways: as a need for change, a preparedness for active participation, recognising the existence of a psychological problem, curiosity or interpersonal attraction (Cartwright & Lerner, 1963). While not being a stable construct, one might nevertheless assume that at least early on during treatment, there is a minimum level of motivation, otherwise the client would immediately discontinue treatment.

Gomes-Schwartz (1978) found a correlation between initial client involvement and success, whereas O'Malley et al (1983) reported the predictive value of involvement, when assessed at the third session. Sloane et al. (1975) reported that in both behavioural and psychoanalytic treatment, those clients who were more active benefited most from treatment. In the Vanderbilt Project comparing therapists and para-professionals, the pattern of results was the same (Strupp & Hadley, 1979), again highlighting the importance of clients' active involvement.

These results indicate that expectancy is related to outcome, particularly when the therapist does not motivate the client to participate actively in treatment.

Self-exploration is considered an essential condition for change in client-centered therapy. Orlinsky and Howard (1986) reviewed 18 studies involving self-exploration and, surprisingly, in the majority of studies, they did not find a correlation between this construct and various measures of treatment outcome. These authors interpreted the negative results as evidence for concluding that self-exploration frequently takes place in both successful and unsuccessful therapies.

Openness and Transfer/Generalization have received comparatively less attention in the literature. Truax and Wittmer (1971) in a review of studies investigating openness, showed that this client characteristic has a positive correlation with treatment outcome. The process of generalizing or inferring from the session to the client's personal environment is a necessary aspect of treatment. This is specifically the case in therapies where self-control procedures have been emphasized to facilitate this process.

Therapist behavioural characteristics—clients' ratings of therapeutic style

Most studies investigating therapist style use the client's rating of therapy as an indicator of therapist helpfulness. In such studies the focus is on the personal quality of the therapist and aspects of the therapeutic relationship. Therapeutic techniques and strategies seem to be of secondary importance even though these are consistently deemed to be the most important aspect of therapeutic change. The characteristics that clients perceive as important and that show a positive relationship with outcome are listed below (Bent, Putnam, Kiesler & Nowicki, 1976; Kaschak, 1978; Llewellyn & Hume, 1979; Murphy, Cramer & Lillie, 1984; Ryan & Gyzynsky, 1971; Sloane, Staples, Whipple & Cristol, 1977; Strupp, Walach & Wogan, 1964):

- a person with whom I can discuss my personal problems and who helps me understand them,
- emotional warmth and understanding,
- a sympathetic and powerful personality,
- the experience of support and comfort,
- offering advice.

Although such reports cover different psychotherapeutic schools, the findings are surprisingly similar. Sloane et al. (1977) and Llewellyn and Hume (1979) obtained client ratings in the comparison of behaviour therapy and psychoanalytic therapy. No substantial differences were reported, thus confirming the importance of the therapeutic relationship as the medium for change. Often therapists and clients differ in their perceptions of therapy: clients tend to emphasise relationship aspects and therapists understandably emphasise clinical techniques (Feifel & Eels, 1963; Kaschak, 1978). Although these retrospective and global ratings of the therapeutic process give little information about specific stages or specific events during therapy, it is possible to extract the qualities of good therapists. The results of these studies consistently identify three dimensions: *empathy/understanding, support and advisement/directiveness*.

Using post-treatment ratings and correlating them with outcome, Boelens and Emmelkamp (1986) noted the consistent relationship between providing a good therapeutic relationship and positive outcome. Although the studies reviewed were essentially behavioural, Gurman (1977) and Orlinsky and Howard (1986), reviewing a different literature, reached the same conclusion. Our brief review will focus on behaviourally oriented studies, because they do not usually emphasise the importance of interpersonal relationship factors.

The results reported by Sloane et al. (1977) indicated that clients receiving behaviour therapy rated their therapists higher on their level of interpersonal contact, accurate empathy and congruence than did clients receiving psychoanalytic treatment. Clients who were liked by their therapists improved their chance of positive change and those who had the most favourable outcome indicated that the interaction with the therapist had been the most helpful aspect of the treatment.

Alexander et al (1976) studied therapists' interpersonal skills in the context of behaviourally oriented family therapy. They report that a global rating of interpersonal skills contributed significantly to the variance in outcome. Similarly, Ford (1978) investigated the relationship between therapists' behaviour during a session and the clients' perception of the quality of the therapeutic relationship. He showed that a nonverbal style characterized by warmth, assurance, honesty, control, relaxation and emotional responsiveness correlated with positive ratings of the relationship.

Rabavilas et al (1979) obtained ratings from descriptions by clients presenting with obsessive-compulsive problems of their therapists' attitudes during exposure treatment. The assessments carried out at a 15-month follow-up showed that respect for the client, understanding and interest were significantly related to outcome. The extent to which the therapist had satisfied the client's dependency needs had a significantly negative correlation with outcome. With regard to the way treatment had been conducted, support, challenging, and explicitness had positive and signficant correlations with outcome, while, in contrast, permissiveness, tolerance and neutrality showed negative correlations.

Comparable results were presented by Schindler et al (1983), who found that couples receiving behavioural marital therapy, and who showed clear improvements at follow-up, rated their therapists as more empathic, directive and active.

Many researchers have used the Relationship Inventory (RI; Barrett-Lennard, 1986; Lietaer, 1976) as a way of measuring therapist characteristics. Hoogduin et al (1988) studied 60 obsessive-compulsive clients treated with exposure and response prevention. They found a significant and positive correlation between outcome and the quality of the therapeutic relationship, as assessed by both clients and therapists.

Emmelkamp and Van der Hout (1983) reported a similar finding for agoraphobics. In most of the studies using the Relationship Inventory, the quality of the therapeutic relationship is measured after the 10th session, when a termination effect may influence the rating. In a second study, reported by Hoogduin et al. (1988), a significant correlation was found after the second session, but this only applied to the clients' ratings of their therapists.

The results from these enquiries, particularly in behaviour therapy, indicate that the quality of the therapeutic relationship in the early phase of treatment can predict outcome. However, it should be noted that these findings are general and do not necessarily reflect microprocesses within therapeutic interactions.

Observer ratings and manipulation of therapist style

Empathy, emotional warmth, and genuinenness These three Rogerian principles have been extensively studied and were reviewed in Chapter 1. There are some relevant studies in behaviour therapy in which the style of the therapist with regard to these conditions was experimentally manipulated. Morris and Suckerman (1974) reported that an emotionally warm and friendly therapist produced greater improvement with systematic desensitization than a cold aloof therapist. Chiappone, McCarey, Piccinin and Schmidtgoessling (1981) compared assertiveness training combined with the Rogerian variables with assertiveness training alone. No differences in outcome were reported, suggesting that effectiveness depends on the nature of the problem and the relevant client behaviour. The question therefore should not be the extent to which a general style of therapy increases success, but rather when specific therapeutic styles are utilized in treatment.

Support Here support refers to encouragement as well as positive feedback. Reinforcement has always been emphasized in behaviour therapy, as shown in studies comparing the different schools of therapy (Brunink & Schroeder, 1979; DeRubeis et al, 1982; Greenwald et al, 1981; Schaap & Suntjens, 1985). In most studies, therapeutic style is rated by clients, but in some cases independent observers have also rated therapists (Bouchard et al, 1980; Truax, 1970).

Directiveness Research correlating directive style and outcome has produced contradictory findings. Beutler, Dunbar and Baer (1980) and Mintz, Luborsky and Auerbach (1971) reported a positive correlation between modest or strong directiveness and treatment success. However, Cooley and Lajoy (1980) and Luborsky et al. (1980) failed to replicate these findings. Experimentally varying therapists' behaviour has also yielded inconsistent findings. Ringler (1977) studied the process of systematic desensitization combined with either rigid or flexible therapist behaviour. Flexible therapists appear to have the most effective and succesful therapeutic approach, suggesting an initial rigid/authoritarian style that gradually changes and becomes more flexible. Ashby, Ford, Guerney and Guerney (1957) instructed therapists to show reflective or directive statements. Although no differences in effectiveness were reported, it appeared that defensiveness and aggression responded favourably to a more reflective style, whereas they increased in response to the directive style. It seems likely therefore, that there is an interaction between therapeutic style and client characteristics.

The studies reviewed thus far have made two important contributions to process research. It has been shown that the quality of the therapeutic relationship can predict outcome. This appears to be the case when the assessment has been carried out early in treatment, highlighting the importance of the initial perceptions of the therapeutic relationship. Secondly, important dimensions have been identified implying that stable behavioural characteristics exert a positive effect on client change and therefore contribute to outcome. This needs to be qualified by noting the contribution made by the type of disturbance, stage of therapy and client behaviour. Therapists do not simply offer good or bad therapeutic relationships, rather they need to assess in what situation, and with what client, particular therapist behaviours produce positive outcomes.

Client and therapist behaviour during therapy

The remaining sections of this chapter examine the results that have emerged from systematically observing client and therapist behaviour. The focus is on discrete behavioural events and their effect on the client-therapist interaction.

Client behaviour: investigating separate categories

Problem description Four studies have offered data on the frequency of this specific behavioural category over the course of treatment. Hill et al. (1983) presented a detailed case description showing a gradual yet noticeable decline in problem description over the course of therapy. Overall, 54% of all client behaviours were rated as descriptions of presenting problems. Snyder (1945) presented an analysis of six cases showing a decrease from 49 to 18%, whereas Hochdörfer et al. (1983) showed that 30% of all client communication involved problem description. Stiles and Sultan (1979) analysed 10 transcripts of sessions from therapists of different schools using the VRM. Irrespective of therapist behaviour, 75% of client activity involved describing feelings and problems.

Discussing plan for change In contrast to the decrease in problem description, Snyder (1945) reported an increase in discussions of plans for change from just 1% at the beginning to 12% at the end of treatment. However, Hill et al. (1983) in their incidental reporting of this category, found that it did not constitute more than 1% of total client activity.

Experiencing and insight This constituted 13% of client activity at the beginning of therapy whereas at the end, it increased to 30% (Hill et al, 1983). Within sessions, there was an increase in the second half of the session. Using a similar category, new orientation, Hochdörfer et al. (1983) reported that overall, this constituted 14% of client communication.

Self-disclosure Stiles et al (1979) analysed 94 short segments from different therapy sessions using the Experiencing Scale devised by Klein, Mathieu, Gendlin and Kiesler (1969) and the VRM system. Disclosure showed the highest correlation on the Experiencing Scale whereas the factual description of a problem (Edification) yielded a negative correlation; similarly, McDaniel, Stiles and McGaughy (1981) reported high correlations between disclosure and self-exploration using the VPS (Gomes-Schwartz, 1978).

Resistant behaviour Snyder (1945) studied resistant behaviour in 27 families in the context of parent training. Two sessions were coded during the initial, middle and end phases of treatment. Interruption, negative attitude and provocation were coded during the initial, middle and end phases of treatment. Interruption, negative attitude and provocation were coded as resistant behaviour. They showed that just nine (33%) of the families exhibited low levels of resistant behaviour. The authors also report a positive correlation between the frequency of this behaviour at the beginning and middle phases of treatment. Successful treatments were characterized by decreases in this behaviour from the beginning to the end of treatment, although the level at the beginning of treatment bore no relationship with later outcome.

Kersten (1987) and Van Bohemen (1987) studied 12 cases of controlled drinking and reported relatively low levels of resistant behaviour (refusal, avoidance, criticism, provocation and resignation), showing an increase in resistant behaviour in the last compared with the first session. This category of behaviour also correlated positively with outcome. This seems to suggest that resistant behaviour should not be considered as a negative aspect of the therapeutic process, but may well indicate that therapy affects clients irrespective of whether they exhibit resistance (Orlinsky & Howard, 1986). Auld and White (1959) compared two experienced with two less experienced psychoanalytic therapists. The experienced therapists were more directive and responded more assuredly towards their resistant clients, whereas the less experienced therapists were more hesitant with their interpretations.

Rejection of interpretation and request for information These are two categories used by Snyder (1945). The first comprised 3% and the latter 5% of all client communication.

Client behaviour: during a single session

Hill et al. (1983) examined the behavioural changes over the course of a session. They reported a decrease in problem description and an increase in self-exploration, insight and silence, indicating that therapy-relevant behaviour tends to occur during the second half of a session. Anchor and Sandler (1973) studied the second session from 35 cases and found that emotional self-disclosure increased as the session progressed and was highest towards the end. Auld and Wilkinson (1973) reported an increase in new experiences and self-observation over time, but this pattern was not evident in psychoanalytic sessions.

Client behaviour: impact on therapist behaviour

The impact of client behaviour on subsequent therapist behaviour was studied by Hochdörfer et al. (1983). Therapists tended to respond to clients' expression of feelings with the relevant reflection of emotional content. In contrast, if the content was more rational, then therapists tended to reciprocate by reflecting the rational content of the exchange. Lee, Hallberg and Harrard (1979), in an analogue study, experimentally varied clients' responses towards those therapist statements containing the reflection of feelings. Results indicated that therapists who experienced contingent verbal or nonverbal reinforcement increased the frequency of those statements. This increase was significant compared to a control group where clients, played by actors, gave noncontingent reinforcement.

Meier and Boivin (1986) analysed segments from 10 sessions identifying conflict solving statements. There was an increase in conflict resolution attempts when statements included a formulation of need and a decrease when statements included a cognitive process. Furthermore, descriptions of positive feelings tended to increase and descriptions of unpleasant feelings decrease when the solution of the conflict became apparent.

In summary, client behaviour appears to be mainly characterized by problem descriptions. As one would expect, this is particularly the case at the beginning of treatment; but over time, as well as during the course of one session, this tends to decrease. The description and exploration of feelings is less evident and constitutes a smaller percentage of client communication. Statements relevant to change, such as discussing change strategies and new insights, comprise a small percentage of individual sessions, though this increases as treatment progresses.

Therapist behaviour

Most researchers have investigated only therapist behaviour (excluding client behaviour), reflecting their interest in identifying the therapist's influence, while ignoring the reciprocal influence occurring within therapeutic dyads. In order to classify the numerous studies, we will draw on those categories most consistent with the schema devised by Elliot et al. (1982b) described in the previous chapter. Our discussion will have three foci: the frequency of each therapist's behaviour, its impact on client behaviour and, where possible, an attempt to suggest when, within sessions, particular behaviours tend to have maximum impact.

Empathy, emotional warmth and understanding Although these classical Rogerian styles are no longer seen as sufficient conditions for positive therapeutic change, all therapeutic schools emphasize them as ways of establishing the therapeutic alliance. The relevant therapist behaviours are labeled as reflection or exploration in the different observational systems (Barkham & Shapiro, 1986). Reflection is defined as therapist statements in which descriptions of the client are repeated or paraphrased and which refer to implied feelings. This could be confused with the interpretation category which is evident by the relatively low inter-observer agreement scores.

As might be expected, therapists from different therapeutic schools show clear differences in the frequency of these statements. Hill et al. (1983), reporting a study of psychoanalytically orientated therapists, showed that only 5% of therapeutic communication involved these Rogerian categories, whereas in studies with client-centred therapists, Hochdörfer et al. (1983) and Snyder (1945) reported frequencies of 29 and 45% respectively.

Frank and Sweetland (1962) studied 160 sessions and reported that clients tend to respond to therapist paraphrasing with new insights. Hochdörfer et al. (1983) also reported that where therapists reflect emotional content, this increases the probability of further client problem descriptions. Hill and Gormally (1977) showed that direct questioning of feelings tends to evoke a higher frequency of expressions of feelings than reflection or reformulation. This was confirmed by Hopkinson et al. (1981) in their study of psychiatric intake sessions, but only if the client had previously talked about feelings. They also found that therapist empathy produced increased client self-disclosure.

Elliott (1979) studied the impact of specific therapist behaviours and found that both reflection and confirmation convey a sense of being understood, although in a later study (Elliot et al, 1982a) both clients and independent observers rated reflection and self-disclosure as not being particularly helpful. Elliott distinguished between two clusters of behaviour: assignment-related and relationship-related. The results indicated that the experience of feeling understood was associated with the relationship-related cluster. The therapist behaviour that contributed to this experience included the Rogerian variables, reinforcement and the therapist's personal impression. Similar results were reported by Barkham and Shapiro (1986); they studied episodes where clients reported that they felt understood, in sessions from the early and later stages. In both stages, reflection, exploration and interpretation were identified as important therapist behaviour, whereas reassurance only led to feeling understood.

It seems that direct questions about feelings may encourage clients to express them. Where the client has already done so, and the therapist wishes to promote more feeling statements, it seems that reflections are an appropriate therapeutic response. Furthermore, reflections are likely to give the client a feeling of being understood, particularly in the early stage of treatment. This supports the beliefs of Johnson and Matross (1977) that empathy and emotional warmth are necessary in gaining the client's trust, though these do not necessarily lead to therapeutic change.

Self-disclosure This category is defined as communicating private and intimate personal information (Jourard, 1971). In everyday interaction, a degree of self-disclosure is considered to be important in establishing interpersonal relationships, and it tends to be reciprocal (Gouldner, 1960). Since client self-disclosure is considered to be an important goal of psychotherapy, one might assume on the basis of this reciprocity that therapists' self-disclosure would lead to client self-disclosure. Some analogue studies indeed lend support to this hypothesis (Jourard & Jaffé, 1970; Pope, 1979; Powell, 1968). However, therapists who disclose about themselves have been seen as sympathetic but at the same time psychologically less stable (Weigel, Dinges, Dyer and Straumfjord, 1972; Wiegel & Warnath, 1968) and more relaxed, albeit weaker (Dies, 1973). The self-disclosure category generally has a low frequency in observational studies, although Barkham and Shapiro (1986) found that therapists using systematic desensitization tended to exhibit much higher rates. The therapeutic situation implies a power relationship, so therapist self-disclosure can undermine therapists' status as experts. Curtis (1982) showed that therapist self-disclosure resulted in lower client empathy and trust and lower perceptions of therapist competence.

Support This category comprises behaviours such as approval/reassurance, confirmation and reinforcement and functions as a source of support and positive feedback. It is therefore of considerable importance in comparing the methods and techniques of contrasting schools of psychotherapy. Snyder (1945) reported that it accounted for 3% of early therapist communication which increased to 10% towards the end of therapy. Similarly, Hill et al. (1983) reported that 3% of total therapist behaviours were coded as support. If minimal support such as recapping is included, it increases to 40%, making this an important category. Similar rates have been reported by Barkham and Shapiro (1986), Kersten (1987) and Van Bohemen (1987), although Hill et al. (1983) have noted that the frequency of support decreases as therapy progresses.

Bandura et al. (1960) found that clients show less aggressive and resistant behaviour towards therapists who show high levels of support and positive feedback. Snyder (1945) showed that support led to the highest contingent frequency of both proposals for change and insights. Several studies have shown its positive impact on the client's experience: Elliott et al. (1982b) found support to be rated as the most helpful therapist behaviour and also that it was used to signal understanding. Although Orlinsky and Howard (1986) stated that support might help but certainly does not harm, the studies seem to suggest that it is at least as important as reflection.

Control and directiveness This category contains those therapist activities that encourage the client to exhibit and practise particular behaviours both during and outside the session and includes instructions, advisements and assignments. It is therefore a characteristic of behaviour therapists, but is used increasingly in other therapeutic approaches (Wogan & Norcross, 1985; Eymael, 1986). Many studies show that clients expect and require directives, and are disappointed if they do not receive them (for a review, see Proctor & Rosen, 1983).

Barkham and Shapiro (1986) reported that control and directiveness account for 4% of therapist behaviour during both the first and fourth sessions, while Hill et al (1983) reported just 1% for direct guidance. These directive statements can contribute to the development of new client perspectives and facilitate the process of problem solving (Elliott et al., 1982b). It is used inconsistently by therapists following a client-centred or psychoanalytic orientation, and even varies within behaviour therapy sessions (flooding versus systematic desensitization); it has been shown to enhance the effectiveness of assertiveness training.

Barkham and Shapiro (1986) distinguished between general advice and instructions. They report a negative correlation between advice and empathy during the first session and low correlations by the fourth. Recommendations about its use can be inferred from both studies by Abramowitz, Abramowitz, Roback and Jackson (1974) and Friedman and Dies (1974), who suggested that externally attributing clients benefit from directive therapies.

Questioning Therapists need to gather information about their clients and regularly do so through questions. Hochdörfer et al. (1983) reported that 14% of therapist activity can be coded as information gathering which elicits both descriptions of feelings and factual information. Lavalle (1977) compared client-centred and behaviourally oriented interview behaviour and found that targeted questioning facilitated goal-directed and change-oriented statements and also had no adverse effect on descriptions of emotional content. Cox, Rutter and Holbrook (1981a,b) were able to show in their analyses of psychiatric intakes that systematic questioning yielded the richest information, whereas multiple questions led to ambiguous answers.

Stiles (1979) reported that 14% of all psychoanalytic therapists' activity could be coded as questions, whereas 3% of client-centred and 21% of Gestalt therapists were coded in this way. Similar trends were given by Schaap and Suntjes (1985). Within behaviour therapy the percentage varied from 6% during systematic desensitization to 20% during a behavioural analysis session.

Some coding systems differentiate between open and closed questions but the rate of occurrence does not change over the course of therapy. During the second half of therapy, clients tend to respond more readily to open questions, often with insight, whereas closed questions tend to be followed by problem description (Barkham & Shapiro, 1986; Hill et al., 1983). Elliott (1979) reported that therapists' intention is best recognized when questions are used, even if they are not seen as necessarily helpful. This is not to suggest that questions should be avoided, given that they have been seen to relate to insight and cognitive restructuring. Similarly, Barkham and Shapiro (1986) noted that open questions are often preceded by instances when clients feel understood. Closed questions yield particular information, thus it is not surprising that clients experience them as unhelpful. The distinction between open and closed questions is essentially their grammatical form. While they both may focus on feelings or contain provocative, confronting or paradoxical elements, their intersubjective effect is clearly different.

Clarification and structuring These serve to structure the therapeutic process (Proctor & Rosen, 1983) and can include providing information about the context of therapy. Hill et al. (1983) reported 10% of all therapist behaviours as attempts to structure sessions with slight increases over the course of treatment. Hochdörfer et al. (1983) found these to comprise just 4%, and Barkham and Shapiro (1986) reported an increase from 8 to 11% from the first to the fourth session. In contrast, Snyder (1945) reported a decrease from 9 to 1% from the beginning to the end of therapy. The sequential analysis carried out by Hochdörfer showed that structuring and clarifications were mainly followed by problem descriptions and to a lesser extent by descriptions of experiences. The case study reported by Hill et al. (1983) showed a high contingent frequency only in regard to problem description. Finally, Elliott et al. (1982b) reported that clarifications after advice and interpretations, were experienced as the most helpful of the therapists' behaviours.

Interpretation This describes how the therapist might move away from the immediate narrative and interpret it therapeutically or make inferences about causal relationships, personality characteristics or other client features. It therefore contains therapist behaviour with differing degrees of complexity and may vary from statements that are similar to clarifications to those where inferences are drawn about unconscious processes. It is not possible to compare studies when the definitions are too varied, a factor that may be more important than differences between therapists from different schools. For example, Sloane et al. (1975) did not find differences in interpretations when comparing psychoanalytic and behaviour therapists.

Hill et al. (1983) reported an increase in interpretations from 10% in the first half to 17% in the second half of therapy, whereas Barkham and Shapiro (1986) reported 7% in the first and 6% in the fourth session. Stiles (1979) showed that almost half of all psychoanalytic and a quarter of all Gestalt interventions were interpretations, while almost none of the client-centred interventions could be coded as such. Schaap and Suntjes (1985) reported 20% for both psychoanalytic and Gestalt therapists, whereas client-centred therapists used interpretations only 5% of the time. Within behaviour therapy, interpretations varied from 3% in the behavioural analysis session to 17% in the flooding session.

Sequential analysis has also been used to study the impact of interpretations on client behaviour and has produced contradictory findings. Hill et al. (1983) noted a significantly reduced frequency in problem description in the first half of therapy that disappears in the second half. Frank and Sweetland (1962) also noted a decreased conditional probability of problem descriptions but an increase in the conditional probability of new insights and understanding following interpretations. Similarly, Hochdörfer et al. (1983) reported an increased probability of experience and rational descriptions of problems. Hopkinson et al (1981) and Auerswald (1974) reported an increased probability of self-disclosure. Other analogue research also reports on the negative effects of interpretation. Kanfer et al. (1960) found that interpretations function as aversive stimuli, and have an inhibitory effect on the communication between the client and therapist. Helner and Jessel (1974) found, in their analogue study, that when students were instructed to rate segments from different videotaped sessions they responded negatively to interpretations. In the study by Auld and White (1959), clients responded contingently with an increase in short responses and recapping, but the authors also reported that interpretations led to increased resistant behaviour. In contrast, Snyder (1945) found that interpretations were usually followed by rejection. Positive effects were reported by Silberschatz, Fretter and Curtis (1986) to the extent that interpretations were delivered appropriately according to psychoanalytic criteria.

A clearer picture emerges from the research investigating the effect of interpretations on the clients' experience. Elliott et al. (1982b) reported that clients rate interpretation as the element that helped them most and, accordingly, it is rated as an event when the client felt understood or developed new insights. These results should be noted with caution, given the different category definitions used by the various observation systems.

Confrontation and criticism This category refers to identifying a contradiction or discrepancy in clients' behaviour or attitude. If the therapist implies a value judgement then the statement is also coded as a criticism. Thus, all therapist behaviours that clients perceive as aversive are coded as critical. Aversive stimulation might be necessary in the course of treatment in order to suggest that the clients change certain problematic behaviours (confrontation) or to point out the negative consequences of not carrying out an assignment. It is unclear whether confrontation and criticism refer to necessary and appropriate therapist behaviour or if they occur out of a sense of helplessness and difficulty in case management. This type of therapist behaviour can easily be construed as punishment and can have a negative effect on outcome (Gustavson et al, 1985). Of course, it is necessary to point out the consequences of unco-operative behaviour which would then be coded as criticism or confrontation.

Hill et al. (1983) reported a 5% frequency for this category and found that it can produce new client insights. Frank and Sweetland (1962), who used a similar category, reported that it led to an increase in both proposals for change and insight. Snyder (1945) noted no criticism or confrontation at the beginning of treatment and 5% at the end of treatment in his analysis of six client-centred therapy cases. Furthermore, he observed that after statements implying criticism or where the client experienced pressure, there was an associated increase in rejection and problem/symptom description.

Silence Thinking and pauses are necessary ingredients in the natural flow of conversation, yet the use of silence as a means of pressuring clients is rejected by most therapists (see Lutz, 1978) and longer silences can be experienced as being aversive. Hill found that silence comprised up to 4% of total therapist time. The positive relationship between silence, insight and new perspectives that has been reported seems to have been attributed to the particular client interaction style. Auld and White (1959) reported that silence was followed by client resistance, whereas Bandura, Lipsher, and Miller (1960) saw silence as an effective way for therapists to deal with aggressive clients and as a means of altering the topic under discussion.

Conclusions and implications

Given the various methodologies and coding schemes that have been used in compiling this review, it is difficult to draw definitive conclusions. The results show both consistencies and contradictions that can be understood as reflecting the range of definitions used, the different therapeutic orientations, the style under investigation and the range of client characteristics. We believe that the consistencies should not be overlooked, despite the availability of inconsistent data.

Globally, there is a change in psychotherapy research from outcome towards process studies. Because this change is so recent, there is as yet little systematic knowledge about process characteristics. Collecting empirically founded results is a time-consuming process, as can be illustrated by an adjoining field of research, marital interaction. Process research in this area was started in the 1970s. And it is after two decades of data-collecting using behaviour observation that we are beginning to understand some of the processes involved in relationship communication and conflict management.

The first phases in process research in psychotherapy will have to consist of collecting descriptions of therapies with differing clients with differing disturbances using valid and reliable instruments. These therapies are only of interest to the extent that process characteristics can be related to outcome of treatment. The second phase will consequently consist of comparing success and failures on particular process features.

In this regard, the suggestions for the design of a process study described in Chapter 6, as well as the process model described in Chapter 2, are quite relevant (see also Schindler, 1990). By standardizing the therapeutic program, the therapeutic processes in the different therapies become comparable. Valid statements can then be made about separate phases in the therapeutic process because similar themes and issues have been handled at the same time in the different therapies.

Continuous video- or audiotaping, as well as coding of all sessions seems sensible and necessary. Only when the total process is captured can statements be made about changes in client or therapist behaviour over the different phases in therapy. Moreover, sequential analysis procedures are needed to study large data sets on a relatively high level of aggregation.

It would, furthermore, be desirable to study the process of psychotherapy in different disorders in order to compare results and to see if they can be replicated and under what conditions. Reliable and valid results on the impact of interaction patterns or strategies of social influence can only be gathered with large numbers of therapies where the symptomatology of the cases is more or less similar and the technical components of treatment are standardized. This latter point is often ignored in process research.

Obviously, process research requires enormous investment. It is for this reason that alternative or complementary strategies of research should be undertaken. One approach consists of the comparison of single case studies, with respect to explicit selected criteria. A comparison of, for instance, the results reported by Kaimer et al. (1989) with those gathered in studies having larger samples shows that both approaches yield essentially the same results. For this reason, single case studies seem appropriate and offer an economic alternative for comparing the validity of results from different disorders.

Another alternative would consist of limiting a study to particular phases in the therapeutic process. If one assumes that the therapeutic relationship is established in the first sessions—self-report studies have repeatedly shown the validity of such an assumption—one could limit the sample to, say, the first three sessions. Important questions then would be: What events lead to a positive experience of the client? Are these events related to the outcome of treatment? In connection with this is the question: What strategy of social influence (as described in Chapters 3 and 4) can be applied by the therapist to achieve this positive experience?

Whatever design is chosen, systematic observation of behaviour appears to be a prerequisite, since the question is: What concrete behavioural elements have to be applied by the therapist? With the present state of the art in process research, it is inevitable that categories are defined behaviourally and whole sessions sampled and coded. This is necessary to ensure enough data for sequential analysis and to circumvent the problem of how to sample excerpts from particular sessions.

It has been put forward that a behavioural coding of the process of therapeutic interaction will not yield anything useful about more complex events in therapy (e.g., Cousins & Power, 1986; Greenberg, 1986a). Nevertheless, it is necessary to gather more knowledge about this level before we make an attempt at formulating hypotheses on a higher level of abstraction.

Sequential analysis of observational data represents the application of a methodology that has been required in the literature for a long time. Consequently, sequential analysis has yielded innovative and well-interpretable results, although some researchers had doubted the usefulness of sophisticated statistical methodology in identifying essential therapeutic interaction patterns (see, for instance, Greenberg, 1986a). Particularly successful and unsuccessful therapies should be compared in this light.

Next to a more quantitative approach in the analysis of the process of psychotherapy, a more qualitative approach can be distinguished. In this approach, episodes are selected on the basis of the experience of the client and therapist. The aim is to study the interactional sequences that lead to positive experiences. Mahrer et al. (1984) have presented an overview of change-relevant episodes.

Ideally, both approaches should be combined. However, at the moment the criteria to arrive at the choice of the change-relevant episode still have to be formulated. Strong discrepancies are reported between clients and therapists in the rating of the extent to which episodes are experienced as helpful or necessary (Elliott, 1979). What is clear, however, is that the experience of the client should carry the most weight and, consequently, should be used as the criterion for the identification of change-relevant episodes. Another problem is that the studies that have been conducted thus far do not succeed in relating the change-relevant episodes to the larger context of the process of the therapy.

The results that have been reported in process research thus far represent the first step in the identification of the effective strategies of social influence. We are beginning to compose a compendium of verbal techniques and a grammar of how to apply these techniques in therapeutic practice. Researchers should try to find a way of empirically testing more complex strategic patterns derived from the practice of communication therapy, such as paradoxical prescriptions, provocation or confrontation. More studies are needed on the impact of such therapeutic techniques.

Strategies of social influence are at least as necessary to achieve change as the application of specific therapeutic techniques. This implies a systematization of what is happening in successful cases. This knowledge will not only enrich the theoretical models used, but will also be of use for the training of therapists. In the end, these strategies will lead to more effective psychotherapy.

The crucial importance of what happens during the first phase of treatment has been pointed out repeatedly. This implies that, during first contact, therapists have to pay close attention to their interpersonal skills and apply these strategically.

The results from different studies on different level of analysis have pointed out the importance of *support*. This behaviour is related to client ratings of a successful session and results in the perception of the therapist as sympathetic, competent and active. This category also is strongly related to consequent cooperative behaviour by the client. The results of the process outcome research shows that therapists who are the least supporting are in the unsuccessful group.

Support, however, does not simply equal reinforcement. It is a complex behavioural category encompassing minimal encouragement, positive feedback and positive labeling, as well as recognition. This therapist behaviour most clearly results in goal orientation and active cooperation. This category therefore seems important in communicating acceptance, as well as increasing the expectancies of clients regarding self-efficiency. In this sense it functions as an antidote against demoralization (Frank, 1973) and builds self-efficacy (Bandura, 1977). This implies that in the case of a reserved or problem-oriented client, therapists have to be more structuring in order to arrive at aspects which they are able to make relevant to treatment and important for change. This also implies that directivity may be an important dimension.

Directivity, the second important dimension, increases structure for the client and increases the likelihood of cooperation. There appears to be an optimum, however. Too much directivity has a negative influence and increases resistance or reactance (Turkat, 1986).

Finally, the third important dimension in therapist behaviour seems to be *empathy*, in its different manifestations. Empathy is necessary to achieve emotional disclosure on the part of the client, because purely factual exploration will not do so. Of course, this has been emphasized repeatedly by the client-centered or person-oriented schools of psychotherapy. Particularly in the initial phase of treatment, such therapist behaviour will entice the client to communicate personal matter, probably mediated by a feeling of trust in the therapist and the therapeutic procedures. It is important to note, however, that these therapist behaviours alone will not lead to change-relevant contributions by the client. They should therefore be combined with behavioural patterns in the other dimensions. Moreover, in the course of treatment it will lose its impact.

Kanfer and Saslow (1974) have already pointed out that during a behaviour analysis, therapists should not only deal with an inventory of the problems and controlling factors. Positive aspects of the person and his or her behaviour are also themes to be discussed. Moreover, therapist behaviour that can be characterized by the dimensions described seems an appropriate strategy for the generation of motivation for change as described by, for instance, Kanfer and Grimm (1980).

A pilot study

To illustrate the foregoing we will end this chapter by describing a pilot study in which we addressed the question: Is it possible to influence the therapeutic relationship at an early stage of treatment, in order to enhance treatment outcome in behaviour therapy?

Fifty-five obsessive clients took part in the study. Group 1 consisted of 30 clients, constituting the experimental group. Efforts were made here to enhance the quality of the therapeutic relationship. Group 2 consisted of 25 clients, constituting the control group. In the treatment of these latter clients no attempt was made to manipulate the therapeutic relationship. The patients of this group had taken part in an earlier study carried out by Hoogduin et al. (1989). The clients were assigned to groups on the basis of the moment they registered for treatment: the first 25 to Group 2, the following 30 to Group 1. The inclusion and exclusion criteria applied were the same for both groups, as was the treatment method. The same instruments of measurement were also used, at the same stages of the therapy. All the patients registered for outpatient treatment, consisting of exposure in vivo and response prevention. The treatment was administered by five therapists; two assigned to the clients in Group 1, and three to those in Group 2. The quality of the therapeutic relationship was assessed after the second and 10th treatment sessions by an independent assessor. Treatment outcome was determined after 10 sessions. Attempts to enhance the quality of the therapeutic relationships of the clients in Group 1 were made between the second and tenth treatment sessions.

The Barrett-Lennard Relationship Inventory (RI; Barrett-Lennard, 1962), adapted by Lietaer (1976) for the Dutch language area, was used to assess the therapeutic relationship. Directly after the second treatment session, the Group 1 clients' RI responses were analysed. Whenever a score on one or more of the items seemed low, the supervisor gave the therapist specific directions for enhancing this aspect of the therapeutic relationship. For each treatment session, the therapist had to indicate on a form designed for this purpose, which directions he had followed (see Fig. 7.1). Since the RI assessment is carried out by an independent assessor, neither the client nor the therapist were aware of the scores.

The directions were arrived at as follows. Approximately 400 descriptions of strategies for getting clients to begin treatment, continue in treatment or take

	Session: 3	4	5	6	7	8	9	10
Make careful use of appreciative remarks								
Show the client that you are pleased to be treating him or her								
Tell the client that he or she is doing his or her best								
Emphasize his or her correct registration of assignments								
Emphasize his or her correct homework assignments								
Compliment the client on his or her perseverence								

Figure 7.1   An illustration for enhancing the quality of the therapeutic relationship

an active part in treatment were collected from the most significant literature in the fields of behavioural therapy, directive therapy, motivation for psychotherapy, compliance and salesmanship. These descriptions were then grouped into 13 categories, each dealing with a different aspect of the therapeutic relationship. (For a detailed account of the categories and examples of motivating strategies, see Schaap & Hoogduin, 1988, and Keijsers, Schaap & Hoogduin, 1990.) When a low score on a particular RI item was recorded, it was decided which category the item best accorded with and which motivating strategies could best be employed. The strategies were then presented in such a way as to provide the therapist with clear, practicable instructions.

Both the clients and therapists in Group 2 (the group in which no attempt was made to influence the therapeutic relationship) assessed the quality of the relationship as having declined during the course of the treatment. An explanation for this could be that the first treatment sessions are primarily used to build up a therapeutic relationship, whilst, by the 10th session, the client and therapist are working together on a process of change. In this later phase the demands they make of each other are greater and the expectations they have of each other's capabilities are more realistic. This can cause them to assess the quality of the therapeutic relationship as having declined.

In Group 1, on the other hand, where attempts were made to manipulate the therapeutic relationship, the quality of the relationship was assessed as having increased between the second and 10th treatment sessions. It was primarily the therapists who felt that the relationship had improved by the second assessment; the client scores remained more or less the same. The instructions geared towards improving the quality of the relationship would seem, therefore, to affect the therapist more than the client. The significant difference in therapist assessment of the therapeutic relationship, found between the groups on second measurement, would seem to indicate that it is possible to influence the relationship in the manner described above.

The improved therapeutic relationship recorded for Group 1 did not actually lead to a significantly better outcome. A positive evaluation of the relationship by the therapist is apparently not enough to ensure more successful treatment. This is not really surprising, since the therapist assessment of the therapeutic relationship accounts for only a part of the variance relating to treatment outcome (approximately 20%). The difference might well have been significant if the Group 1 patient assessment of the relationship had also increased.

A number of methodological problems make it impossible to draw clear conclusions from the above findings. Firstly, the results are based on a small sample and the therapists were not the same for both groups. Secondly, the directions for improving the quality of the therapeutic relationship were based on the very instrument of measurement used for determining any improvement in it. In future research, a parallel instrument of measurement will have to be used to determine the improvement in the quality of the relationship. Thirdly, the question remains as to what extent the improvement in the quality of the relationship in Group 1 can be ascribed to the specific interventions made in order to enhance the quality of the therapeutic relationship, and to what extent was it simply due to the extra attention paid to client–therapist interaction in this group as part of the study design. In order to control for this effect in a future study, clients would have to be assigned at random to two groups, with therapists in the experimental group being given directions for improving the therapeutic relationship, and therapists in the control group being given instructions, for example, on precise application of treatment techniques. Treatment for both groups would have to be the same in all other respects. The expectation would be that clients and therapists dissatisfied with the therapeutic relationship at the beginning of the treatment would gain more from directions for improving the relationship than from instructions about treatment techniques.

In the study presented here, the therapists in particular felt an improvement in the therapeutic relationship. They had made a conscious effort to enhance their relationship with clients and this may account, in part, for the higher therapist assessment score at the second measurement. It may also be that clients give a higher evaluation of the therapeutic relationship when motivated to work towards creating a good relationship. An independent assessor could, for example, tell clients that research has linked favourable treatment outcome to good understanding between client and therapist and that it could therefore be in their interest to work towards developing a sound relationship.

Finally, the questionnaire employed, the RI, may be a limiting factor in this study. This inventory is based on the principles from client-centred therapy and contains items that are indicators of the therapeutic conditions: 'empathy', 'genuineness', 'unconditional acceptance' and 'positive regard'. These are important aspects of the therapeutic relationship, but other, equally important, relationship variables were missing from the study: the therapist as expert, as a helper during change and as a model (Frank, 1973; Strong & Matross, 1973; Strong & Claiborn, 1982).

In spite of these problems, we consider this study one example of a research study in the vein of the process model given in this book. Further research will be needed to determine whether the above findings have any validity. Given the fact that a quarter of patients with obsessive-compulsive neurosis still do not benefit from treatment (as is undoubtedly the case for other disorders as well) (Emmelkamp, 1982; Marks, 1987; Hoogduin & Duivenvoorden, 1988), research in this area is called for.

Conclusion

Research on the different schools of psychotherapy, as practised, presents a picture which provides evidence for the importance of common factors. The emphasis on common factors is often falsely associated with eclecticism and a mere combination of often incompatible ingredients. The concept of common factors represents, however, a meta-model that describes the mechanism valid for all forms of psychotherapy. The further study of these factors contributes to a better understanding of the therapeutic process and at the same time helps to create a stronger connection between research and practice. One of the common factors in the healing practice of psychotherapy, is the client-therapist or therapeutic relationship. Within behavioural psychotherapy, effectiveness of treatment techniques have received more emphasis than the conditions under which these techniques are taught.

With the introduction of social psychological principles in behavioural psychotherapy, a theoretical framework became available that enabled the description and explanation of the social aspects of the therapeutic relationship. The social psychology literature on persuasion examined earlier indicates some of the avenues that can be explored in managing the therapeutic relationship and its effectiveness in bringing about change. The social psychological model fills a theoretical gap in the conceptualization of therapeutic change, explaining the impact of the psychotherapeutic relationship on the client. Change takes place within clients, and the social interaction within psychotherapy provides the conditions for the consequent learning processes.

The next step was the operationalization of specific strategies of social influence; of empirically founded advisements for therapists on how to handle particular clients. In the second part of this volume we have tried to fill this gap by turning to clinical practice. Analysis of a great number of specific strategies to motivate clients to change yielded a scheme that fits well into the social psychological conceptualization of the power of the therapist to influence clients. The scheme is presented here again:

Emphasizing expertise

The therapist mobilizes trust in himself or herself as a person The therapist presents him or herself as a competent, experienced and reliable person, and increases clients' expectation that their problems will be solved.

The therapist promotes trust in the therapeutic procedures The therapist presents a credible formulation of the presenting problem and a logical explanation of the effective components of the therapeutic procedures.

The therapist gives information At the onset of treatment, the therapist provides the client with information about the therapy, the procedures and their respective roles.

Enhancing attraction

The therapist accepts the client unconditionally The therapist accepts the client, warmly affirms him or her as a person and takes him or her seriously.

The therapist is courteous The therapist treats the client appropriately in a courteous manner, which increases the attraction of the therapeutic relationship.

The therapist empathizes with the client The therapist is empathic, interested and enabling, which is expressed in attentive listening as well as in pacing.

Establishing a working alliance

The therapist encourages active participation The therapist encourages the client to adopt an active and participating attitude towards therapy or specific assignments.

The therapist applies pressure The therapist maintains the therapeutic tempo by creating agreements or contracts by which the client feels an obligation to participate in the negotiation.

The therapist involves a third party A positive or participating client attitude is induced by involving a significant other.

Helping with the process of change

The therapist "endorses" the treatment procedures The therapist tailors the treatment plans to the client's needs and preferences by emphasizing the client's strong points and by matching interventions with client characteristics.

The therapist gives support The therapist strengthens the client's self-confidence by directing attention to the positive change that occurs and the experiences of learning that are involved.

The therapist offers help The therapist gives advice and helps in managing problems and makes problems "solvable".

Utilizing reactance

The therapist utilizes reactance The therapist copes with the client's uncooperative behaviour by altering the pattern of interaction or using it differently.

To be able to indicate the type of intervention, i.e., the specific therapist behaviour, for a specific problem with a specific client, much empirical data must still be gathered. In Chapters 6 and 7, we have tried to present an impression of the state of the art in this research. We have pointed out the problems that researchers face, the solutions that have been reached by developing different instruments, and the results that have been obtained. The type of research needed must proceed in a number of phases. The first phase in process research in psychotherapy should consist of collecting descriptions of therapy with a variety of clients with different disturbances using valid and reliable instruments. In the second phase a comparison of success and failures of particular process features should be made. Furthermore, it would be desirable to study the process of psychotherapy for different disorders in order to compare results that attempt replication and investigate the common and differing conditions. Another approach would consist of limiting a study to particular phases in the therapeutic process, in particular the first sessions in which the stage is set for therapeutic change to occur.

The crucial importance of what happens during the first therapy sessions has been pointed out repeatedly. This implies, and this may be the main lesson from this volume, that therapists during their first contact with a client have to assess the motivation of the client for treatment as well as their interpersonal style. Then, therapists will have to pay close attention to their own interpersonal skills and apply these strategically in order to prevent dropout and to create a climate in which clients are "seduced" to try out new behaviours. Some "interpersonal strategies", e.g. support, directivity and empathy, have been systematically studied. If we compare them with the scheme presented above, we immediately see that they constitute only a small sample of the strategies labelled there. Chapters 3–5 describe the more specific therapist behaviours in these categories. The point is that this scheme can be used as a heuristic scheme to generate therapist interpersonal behaviours for solving reasonably specific problems. Of course, it is suggested that these behaviours are adapted to the specific client. In that sense, psychotherapy, including behavioural psychotherapy, has to be *client-centred*. By the same token, the scheme represents a different research approach. Instead of studying the specific effect of each strategy, even if this were feasible, we make use of systematized clinical intuition and experience to find out which solution belongs to which problem. The resulting "match" can then be studied in more empirical investigations.

References

Abramowitz, C.V., Abramowitz, S.I., Roback, H.B. & Jackson, C. (1974). Differential effectiveness of directive and nondirective group therapies as a function of client internal-external control. *Journal of Consulting and Clinical Psychology*, **42**, 849–853.

Acosta, F.X. (1980). Self-described reasons for premature termination from psychotherapy by Mexican-American, Black American and Anglo-American patients. *Psychological Reports*, **47**, 435–443.

Alexander, J.F., Barton, C., Schiavo, S. & Parsons, B.V. (1976). Systems-behavioral intervention with families of delinquents: Therapist characteristics, family behavior and outcome. *Journal of Consulting and Clinical Psychology*, **44**, 656–664.

Alexander, L.B. & Luborsky, L. (1986). The Penn Helping Alliance Scales. In L.S. Greenberg & W.M. Pinsof (Eds.) *The psychotherapeutic process: A research handbook*. New York: Guilford.

Allison, P.D. & Liker, J.K. (1982). Analyzing sequential categorical data on dyadic interaction: A comment on Gottman. *Psychological Bulletin*, **91**, 393–403.

American Psychiatric Association (1987). *Diagnostic and statistical manual of mental disorders*, 3rd Edition, Revised. Washington, DC: APA.

Anchor, K.N. & Sandler, H.M. (1973). *Psychotherapy sabotage and avoidance of self-disclosure*. Reprints from the Proceedings of the 81st Annual Convention of the APA, 483–484. New York: Americal Psychological Association.

Appelbaum, A. (1972). A critical re-examination of the concept Motivation for Change in psychoanalytic treatment. *International Journal of Psychoanalysis*, **53**, 51–59.

Apple, W., Streeter, L.S. & Kraus, S.M. (1979). Effects of pitch and speech rate on personal characteristics. *Journal of Personality and Social Psychology*, **37**, 715–725.

Arentewicz, G. & Schmidt, G. (1980), *Sexuell gestörte Beziehungen: Konzept und Technik der Paartherapie*. [Sexually disturbed relationships: Concept and technique of the partner therapy] Berlin: Springer.

Arrindell, W.A. & Emmelkamp, P.M.G. (1985). Psychological profile of the spouse of the female agoraphobic patient: Personality and symptoms. *British Journal of Psychiatry*, **146**, 405–414.

Arrindell, W.A. & Ettema, J.H.M. (1986), *SCL-90: Handleiding bij een multidimensionele psychopathologie-indicator*. [SCL-90: Manual of a multidimensional psychopathology indicator] Lisse: Swets & Zeitlinger.

Ashby, J.D., Ford, D.H, Guerny, B.G. & Guerny, L.F. (1957). Effects on clients of a reflective and leading type of psychotherapy. *Psychological Monographs*, 453, 71.

Auerswald, M.C. (1974). Differential reinforcing power of restatement and interpretation on client production of affect. *Journal of Counseling Psychology*, 21, 9–14.

Auld, F. & Whyte, A.M. (1959). Sequential dependencies in psychotherapy. *Journal of Abnormal and Social Psychology*, 58, 100–104.

Auld, F. & Wilkinson, W.C. (1973). *Openess and awareness of communications during psychotherapy*. Reprints from the Proceedings, 81st Annual Convention, APA, 487–488. New York: American Psychological Association.

Badura, H.O. (1975). Die Beurteilung von Leidensdruck und bewusster Motivation für Psychotherapie aus dem Erstinterview. [The assessment of suffering and conscious motivation for psychotherapy from the initial interview] *Psychotherapie und Medizinische Psychologie*, 25, 198–202.

Badura, H.O. (1976). Presentation of factors about the indication and suitability for psychotherapy using path analysis. *Nervenartzt*, 47, 232–235.

Baekeland, F. & Lundwall, L. (1975). Dropping out of treatment: A critical review. *Psychological Bulletin*, 82, 738–783.

Bandura, A. (1971). *Psychological modeling*. Chicago: Aldine.

Bandura, A. (1977). Self-efficacy: Toward a unifying theory of behavioral change. *Psychological Review*, 84, 191–215.

Bandura, A., Lipsher, D.H. & Miller, P.E. (1960). Psychotherapists's approach–avoidance reactions to patients' expressions of hostility. *Journal of Consulting Psychology*, 24, 1–8.

Barker, S.L., Funk, S.C. & Houston, B.K. (1988). Psychological treatment versus nonspecific factors: A meta-analysis of conditions that engender comparable expectations for improvement. *Clinical Psychology Review*, 8, 579–594.

Barkham, M. & Shapiro, D.A. (1986). Counselor verbal response modes and experience empathy. *Journal of Counseling Psychology*, 33, 3–10.

Barrett-Lennard, G.T. (1962). Dimensions of therapist response and causal factors in therapeutic personality change. *Psychological Monographs*, 562, 76.

Barrett-Lennard, G.T. (1986). The Relationship Inventory now: Issues and advances in theory, method and use. In L.S. Greenberg & W.M. Pinsof (Eds.), *The psychotherapeutic process: A research handbook*. New York: Guilford.

Becker, M.H. & Green, L.W. (1975). A family approach to compliance with medical treatment: A selective review of the literature. *International Journal of Health Education*, 18, 173–182.

Becker, M.H. & Maiman, L.A. (1980). Strategies for enhancing patient compliance. *Journal of Community Health*, 6, 113–135.

Beier, E.G. (1966). *The silent language of psychotherapy: Social reinforcement of unconscious process*. Chicago: Aldine.

Bekkers, A. & Schaap, C.P.D.R. (1985). Extratherapeutische gebeurtenissen. [Extratherapeutic events] *Tijdschrift voor Psychotherapie*, 12, 279–293.

Benbenishty, R. (1987). Gaps between expectations and perceived reality of therapists and clients. *Journal of Clinical Psychology*, 43, 231–236.

Benjamin, L.S. (1974). Structural analysis of social behavior. *Psychological Review*, 81, 392–425.

Benjamin, L.S. (1979). Use of structural analysis and social behavior (SASB) and Markov chains to study dyadic interactions. *Journal of Abnormal Psychology*, 88, 303–319.

Benjamin, L.S. (1982). Use of structural analysis of social behavior (SASB) to guide interventions in psychotherapy. In J. Anchin & D. Kiesler (Eds.), *Handbook of interpersonal psychotherapy*. New York: Academic Press.

Bennun, I., Hahlweg, K., Schindler, L. & Langlotz, M. (1986). Therapist's and client's perceptions in behavior therapy: The development and cross-cultural analysis of an assessment instrument. *British Journal of Clinical Psychology*, 25, 275–285.

Bennun, I. & Schindler, L. (1988). Therapist and patient factors in the behavioral treatment of phobic patients. *British Journal of Clinical Psychology*, 27, 145–150.

Bent, R.J., Putnam, D.G., Kiesler, D.J. & Nowicki, S. (1976). Correlates of successful and unsuccessful psychotherapy. *Journal of Consulting and Clinical Psychology*, 44, 149.

Berelson, B. (1952). *Content analysis in communication research*. Glencoe: Free Press.

Beutler, L.E., Crago, M. & Arizmendi, T.G. (1986). Research on therapist variables in psychotherapy. In S.L. Garfield & A.E. Bergin (Eds.), *Handbook of psychotherapy and behavior change*. New York: Wiley.

Beutler, L.E., Dunbar, P.W. & Baer, P.E. (1980). Individual variation among therapists' perception of patients, therapy process and outcome. *Psychiatry*, 43, 205–210.

Blanchard, E.D., Andrasik, F., Neff, D.F., Saunders, N.L., Arena, J.G., Pallmeyer, T.P., Teders, S.J. & Jurisch, S.E. (1983). Four process studies in the behavioral treatment of chronic headache. *Behavior Research and Therapy*, 21, 209–220.

Blaser, A. (1981). Will ich diesen Patienten selbst behandeln? [Do I want to treat this patient myself?] *Schweizerische Zeitschrift für Psychologie*, 40, 132–140.

Borgeest, B. (1958). *Verkoopgesprekken*. [Sale interviews] Den Haag: N.V. Maandblad Succes.

Bouchard, M.A., Wright, J., Mathieu, M., Lalonde, F., Bergeron, G. & Toupin, J. (1980). Structured learning in teaching therapists social skills training: Acquisition, maintainance and impact on client outcome. *Journal of Consulting and Clinical Psychology*, 48, 491–502.

Bradac, J.J., Brower, J.W. & Courtright, J.A. (1979). Three language variables in communication research: Intensity, immediacy and diversity. *Human Communication Research*, 5, 257–269.

Brehm, S.S. (1976), *The application of social psychology to clinical practice*. New York: Wiley.

Brehm, S.S. & Smith, T.W. (1986). Social psychology approaches to psychotherapy and behavior change. In S.L. Garfield & A.E. Bergin (Eds.), *Handbook of psychotherapy and behavior change*. New York: Wiley.

Brinkman, W. (1978). Het gedragtherapeutisch proces. [The behaviourtherapeutic process] In J.W.G. Orlemans (Ed.), *Handboek Gedragstherapie*, Deel A. [Handbook Behaviour therapy, Part A] Deventer: Van Loghum Slaterus.

Brunink, S. & Schroeder, H.E. (1979). Verbal therapeutic behavior of expert psychoanalytically oriented, Gestalt and behavior therapists. *Journal of Consulting and Clinical Psychology*, 47, 567–574.

Cacioppo, J.T., Petty, R.E. & Stoltenberg, C.D. (1985). Processes of social influence: The elaboration likelihood model of persuasion. In Kendall, P. (Ed.), *Advances in cognitive–behavioral research and practice* (Vol. 4). New York: Academic Press.

Cappella, J.H. & Street, R.L., Jr. (1985). Introduction: A functional approach to the structure of communicative behavior. In R.L. Street Jr. & J.H. Cappella (Eds.), *Sequence and pattern in communicative behavior*. London: Edward Arnold.

Carkhuff, R. (1969). *Helping and human relations: A primer for lay and professional helpers. Vol 1: Selection and training*. New York: Holt–Rinehart–Winston.

Carson, R.C. (1969). *Interaction concepts of personality*. Chicago: Aldine.

Cartwright, D. (Ed.) (1959). *Studies in social power*. Ann Arbor: The University of Michigan.

Cartwright, R.D. & Lerner, B. (1963). Empathy, need to change, and improvement with psychotherapy. *Journal of Consulting Psychology*, 27, 138–144.

Caspar, F.M. & Grawe, K. (1981). Widerstand in der Verhaltenstherapie. [Resistance in behaviour therapy] In H. Petzold (Ed.), *Widerstand: Ein strittiges Konzept in der Psychotherapie.* [Resistance: A controversial concept in psychotherapy] Paderborn: Junfermann.

Chadwick-Jones, J.K. (1976). *Social exchange theory: Its structure and influence in social psychology.* New York: Academic Press.

Chamberlain, P., Patterson, G., Reid, J., Kavanagh, K. & Forgatch, M. (1984). Observation of client resistance. *Behavior Therapy*, 15, 144–155.

Chiappone, D., McCarrey, M., Piccinin, S. & Schmidtgoessling, N. (1981). Relationship of client-perceived facilitative conditions on outcome of behaviorally oriented assertive training. *Psychological Reports*, 49, 251–256.

Claiborn, C.D., Ward, S.R. & Strong, S.R. (1981). Effects of congruence between counselor interpretations and client beliefs. *Journal of Counseling Psychology*, 28, 101–109.

Cooley, E.J. & Lajoy, R. (1980). Therapeutic relationship and improvement as perceived by clients and therapists. *Journal of Clinical Psychology*, 36, 562–570.

Cooper, J. & Axsom, D. (1982). Cognitive dissonance and psychotherapy. In G. Weary & A. Mirels (Eds.), *Emerging integrations of clinical and social psychology.* New York: Oxford University Press.

Corrigan, J.D., Dell, D.M., Lewis, K.N. & Schmidt, L.D. (1980). Counseling as a social influence process: A review. *Journal of Counseling Psychology Monograph*, 27, 395–441.

Cousins, P.C. & Power, T.G. (1986). Quantifying family process: Issues in the analysis of interaction sequences. *Family Process*, 25, 89–105.

Cox, A., Hopkins, K. & Rutter, M. (1981). Psychiatric interviewing techniques. II. Naturalistic study: Eliciting factual information. *British Journal of Psychiatry*, 138, 283–291.

Cox, A., Rutter, M. & Holbrook, D. (1981a). Psychiatric interviewing techniques. V. Experimental study: Eliciting factual information. *British Journal of Psychiatry*, 139, 29–37.

Cox, A., Rutter, M. & Holbrook, D. (1981b). Psychiatric interviewing techniques. VI. Experimental study: Eliciting feelings. *British Journal of Psychiatry*, 139, 144–152.

Cross, D.G. & Warren, C.E. (1984). Environmental factors associated with continuers and terminators in adult outpatient psychotherapy. *British Journal of Medical Psychology*, 57, 363–369.

Curtis, J.M. (1982). The effect of therapist self-disclosure on patient's perceptions of empathy, competence and trust in an analogue psychotherapeutic interaction. *Psychotherapy: Theory, Research and Practice*, 19, 54–62.

Dabbs, J.M. (1969). *Similarity of gestures and interpersonal influence.* Proceedings of the 77th Annual Convention of the APA, 6, 337–338. New York: American Psychological Association.

Davanloo, H. (Ed.) (1978). *Basic principles and techniques in short-term dynamic psychotherapy.* New York: Spectrum Publications.

Davison, G.L. (1973). Counter-control in behavior modification. In L.A. Hammerlynck, L.C. Handy & E.J. Hash (Eds.), *Behavior change.* Champain: Research Press.

DeRubeis, R.J., Hollon, S.D., Evans, M.D. & Bemis, K.M. (1982). Can psychotherapies for depression be discriminated? A systematic investigation of cognitive therapy and interpersonal therapy. *Journal of Consulting and Clinical Psychology*, 50, 744–756.

DeVoge, J.T. & Beck, S. (1978). The therapist–client relationship in behavior therapy. In M. Hersen, R.M. Eisler & P.M. Miller (Eds.), *Progress in Behavior Modification*, (Vol. 4), pp. 203–249. New York: Academic Press.

Dean, S.I. (1958). Treatment of the reluctant client. *American Psychologist*, **13**, 627–630.

Derogatis, L.R. (1977). *SCL-90: Administration, scoring and procedure manual.* Baltimore MD: Clinical Psychometrics Research Unit, Johns Hopkins University School of Medicine.

Dhaenens, R., Schaap, C., De Mey, H. & Näring, G. (1989). Therapietrouw en Essentiële Hypertensie. [Compliance and Essential Hypertension] *Gedrag en Gezondheid*, **17**, 107–114.

Dies, R.R. (1973). Group therapist self-disclosure: An evaluation by clients. *Journal of Counseling Psychology*, **20**, 344–348.

Dixon, D.N. (1986). Client resistance and social influence. In F.J. Dorn (Ed.), *Social influence processes in counseling and psychotherapy*. Springfield: C.C. Thomas.

Dollard, J. & Miller, N.E. (1950). *Personality and Psychotherapy*. New York: McGraw-Hill.

Donnan, H.H. & Mitchell, H.D. (1979). Preferences for older versus younger counselors among a group of elderly persons. *Journal of Counseling Psychology*, **26**, 514–518.

Dorn, F.J. (1986). *The social influence process in counseling and psychotherapy*. Springfield: Thomas.

Duckro, P., Beal, D. & George, C. (1979). Research on the effects of disconfirmed client role expectations in psychotherapy: A critical review. *Psychological Bulletin*, **86**, 260–275.

Durlak, J.A. (1979). Comparative effectiveness of paraprofessionals and professional helpers. *Psychological Bulletin*, **86**, 80–92.

Elliott, R. (1979). How clients perceive helper behaviors. *Journal of Counseling Psychology*, **26**, 285–294.

Elliott, R. (1983). Fitting process research to the practicing psychotherapist. *Psychotherapy*, **20**, 47–55.

Elliott, R. (1984). A discovery-oriented approach to significant change events in psychotherapy: Interpersonal process recall and comprehensive process analysis. In L. Rice & L. Greenberg (Eds.), *Change episodes*. New York: Guilford.

Elliott, R. (1986). Interpersonal Process Recall as a psychotherapeutic process research method. In L.L. Greenberg & W.M. Pinsof (Eds.), *The psychotherapeutic process: A research handbook*. New York: Guilford.

Elliott, R., Barker, C.B., Caskey, N. & Pistrang, N. (1982a). Differential helpfulness of counselor verbal response modes. *Journal of Counseling Psychology*, **29**, 354–361.

Elliott, R., Hill, C., Stiles, W.B., Friedlander, M.L., Mahrer, A.R. & Margison, F.R. (1987). Primary therapist response modes: Comparison of six rating systems. *Journal of Consulting and Clinical Psychology*, **55**, 218–223.

Elliott, R., Stiles, W.B., Shiffman, S., Barker, C.B., Burstein, B. & Goodman, G. (1982b). The empirical analysis of help-intended communications: Conceptual framework and recent research. In T.A. Wills (Ed.), *Basis processes in helping relationships*. New York: Academic Press.

Emmelkamp, P.M. (1982). *Phobic and obsessive–compulsive disorders: Theory, research and practice*. New York: Plenum.

Emmelkamp, P.M. & Foa, E.B. (1983). Failures are a challenge. In E.B. Foa & P.M.G. Emmelkamp (Eds.), *Failures in behavior therapy*. New York: Wiley.

Emmelkamp, P.M. & Ultee, K.A. (1974). A comparison of successive approximation and self-observation in the treatment of agoraphobia. *Behavior Therapy*, **5**, 606–613.

Emmelkamp, P.M. & Van der Hout, A. (1983). Failure in treating agoraphobia. In E.B. Foa & P.M.G. Emmelkamp (Eds.), *Failures in behavior therapy*. New York: Wiley.

Engel, K. & Wilms, H. (1986). Therapy motivation in Anorexia Nervosa: Theory and first empirical results. *Psychotherapy and Psychosomatics*, **46**, 161–170.

Eymael, J. (1986). *A comparison of client-centered therapy and behavior therapy*. Doctoral Dissertation, University of Nijmegen.

Falloon, I.R.H., Boyd, J.L., McGill. C.W. (1984). *Behavioural family management of mental illness: Enhancing family coping in community care*. New York: Guilford.

Feifel, H. & Eels, J. (1963). Patients and therapist assess the same psychotherapy. *Journal of Consulting Psychology*, **27**, 310–318.

Feldman, M.P. (1976). Social psychology and the behavior therapies. In M.P. Feldman & A. Broadhurst (Eds.), *Theoretical and experimental bases of the Behavior Therapies*. New York: Wiley.

Festinger, L. (1954). A theory of social comparison processes. *Human Relations*, **7**, 117–140.

Fiedler, F. (1950). The concept of an ideal therapeutic relationship. *Journal of Consulting Psychology*, **14**, 239–245.

Fiedler, P. (1974). Gesprächsführung bei verhaltenstherapeutischen Explorationen. [Conversing in behaviourtherapeutic exploration] In D. Schulte (Ed.), *Diagnostik in der Verhaltenstherapie*. [Diagnostics in behaviour therapy] München: Urban & Schwarzenberg.

Fiester, A. & Rudestan, K. (1975). A multivariate analysis of the early dropout process. *Journal of Consulting and Clinical Psychology*, **43**, 528–535.

Fiske, D.W. (1977). Methodological issues in research on the psychotherapist. In A.S. Gurman & A.M. Razin (Eds.), *Effective psychotherapy*. Oxford: Pergamon.

Foa, E.B. & Foa, U.G. (1980). Resource theory: Interpersonal behavior as exchange. In K.J. Gergen, M.S. Greenberg & R.H. Willis (Eds.), *Social exchange: Advances in theory and research*. New York: Plenum.

Ford, J. (1978). Therapeutic relationship in behavior therapy: An empirical analysis. *Journal of Consulting and Clinical Psychology*, **46**, 1302–1314.

Foster, S.L. & Cone, J.D. (1986). Design and use of direct observation procedures. In A.R. Ciminero, K.S. Calhoun & E.H. Adams (Eds.), *Handbook of behavioral assessment*. New York: Wiley.

Frank, J.D. (1973). *Persuasion and healing*, 2nd Edition. Baltimore: Johns Hopkins University Press.

Frank, J. D. (1982). Biofeedback and the placebo. *Biofeedback and self-regulation*, **7**, 449–460.

Frank, J.D. (1985). Shared therapeutic features of psychotherapies. In P. Pichot, P. Berner, R. Wolf & K. Thau (Eds.), *Psychiatry: The state of the art*. New York: Plenum.

Frank, G.H. & Sweetland, A. (1962). A study of the process of psychotherapy: The verbal interaction. *Journal of Consulting Psychology*, **26**, 135–138.

Freedman, J. & Fraser S.C. (1966). Compliance without pressure: The foot-in-the-door technique. *Journal of Personality and Social Psychology*, **4**, 195–202.

French, J.R.P., Jr & Raven, B. (1959). The bases of social power. In D. Cartwright (Ed.) *Studies in Social Power*. Ann Arbor: University of Michigan Press.

Friedlander, M.L. (1982). Counseling discourse as a speech event: Revision and extension of the Hill Counselor Verbal Response Category System. *Journal of Counseling Psychology*, **29**, 425–429.

Friedman, M.L. & Dies, R.R. (1974). Reactions of internal and external test-anxious students to counseling and behavior therapies. *Journal of Consulting and Clinical Psychology*, **42**, 921.

Fuller, F. & Hill, C.E. (1985). Counselor and helper perceptions of counselor intentions in relation to outcome in a single counseling session. *Journal of Counseling Psychology*, **32**, 329–338.

Garfield, S.L. (1981). Evaluating the psychotherapies. *Behavior Therapy*, **12**, 295–307.

Garfield, S.L. (1986). Research on client variables in psychotherapy. In S.L. Garfield & A.E. Bergin (Eds.), *Handbook of psychotherapy and behavior change*. New York: Wiley.

Garfield, S.L., Affleck, D. & Muffly, R. (1963). A study of psychotherapeutic interaction and continuation in psychotherapy. *Journal of Consulting and Clinical Psychology*, **19**, 473–478.

Garfield, S. & Bergin, A. (1986). *Handbook of psychotherapy and behavior change*. New York: Wiley.

Gendlin, E.T. (1973). Experiential psychotherapy. In R. Corsini (Ed.), *Current psychotherapies*. Itaska: Peacock.

Giles, H. & Powesland, P.F. (1975). *Speech style and social evaluation*. London: Academic Press.

Goldfried, M.R. (1982). Resistance and clinical behavior therapy. In P.L. Wachtel (Ed.), *Resistance, psychodynamic and behavioural approaches*. New York, Plenum.

Goldstein, A. (1962). *Therapist and patient expectancies in psychotherapy*. New York: Macmillan.

Gomes-Schwartz, B. (1978). Effective ingredients in psychotherapy: Prediction of outcome from process variables. *Journal of Consulting and Clinical Psychology*, **46**, 1023–1035.

Gomes-Schwartz, G. & Schwartz, J.M. (1978). Psychotherapy process variables distinguishing the "inherently helpful" person from the professional psychotherapist. *Journal of Consulting and Clinical Psychology*, **46**, 196–197.

Goodman, G. & Dooley, D. (1976). A framework for help-intended communication. *Psychotherapy*, **13**, 106–117.

Gottman, J.M. (1979). *Marital interaction: Experimental investigations*. New York: Academic Press.

Gouldner, A.W. (1960). The norm of reciprocity: A preliminary statement. *American Sociological Review*, **25**, 161–178.

Gouwe, W.F.K. (1961). *Welke zieken zoeken een magnetiseur?* [Which patients consult a magnetiser?] Hilversum Nederlandse Werkgroep Paragnosten.

Greenberg, L.S. (1986a). Change process research. *Journal of Consulting and Clinical Psychology*, **54**, 4–9.

Greenberg, L.S. (1986b). Research strategies. In L.S. Greenberg & W.M. Pinsof (Eds.), *The psychotherapeutic process: A research handbook*. New York: Guilford.

Greenberg, L.S. & Pinsof, W.M. (1986). Process research: Current trends and future perspectives. In L.S. Greenberg & W.M. Pinsof (Eds.), *The therapeutic process: A research handbook*. New York: Guilford.

Greenspan, M. & Kulish, N.M. (1985). Factors in long-term psychotherapy. *Psychotherapy*, **22**, 1, 75–82.

Greenwald, D.P., Kornblith, S.J., Hersen, M., Bellack, A.S. & Himmelhoch, J.M. (1981). Differences between social skills and psychotherapists in treating depression. *Journal of Consulting and Clinical Psychology*, **49**, 757–759.

Gurman, A.S. (1977). The patient's perception of the therapeutic relationship. In A.S. Gurman & A.M. Razin (Eds.), *Effective psychotherapy: A research handbook*. New York: Pergamon.

Gustavson, B., Jansson, L., Jerremalm, A. & Öst, L.G. (1985). Therapist behavior during exposure treatment of agoraphobia. *Behavior Modification*, **9**, 491–504.

Hahlweg, K. (1981). Die Bedeutung der Therapeutenvariable in der Verhaltenstherapie. [The significance of the therapist variable in behaviour therapy] In J.C.

Brengelmann (Ed.), *Entwicklung der Verhaltenstherapie in der Praxis.* [Development of behaviour therapy in practice] IFT Texte. Munich: Röttger, 6.

Hahlweg, K. & Jacobson, N.S. (Eds) (1984). *Marital interaction: Analysis and modification.* New York: Guilford.

Hahlweg, K., Langlotz, M. & Schindler, L. (1983). *Rating of the therapist's behavior by the client: Relationship with outcome.* Munich: Max Planck Institute for Psychiatry.

Hahlweg, K., Reisner, L., Kohli, G., Vollmer, M., Schindler, L. & Revenstorf, D. (1984). Development and validity of a new system to analyse interpersonal communication (KPI). In K. Hahlweg & N. Jacobson (Eds.), *Marital interaction: Analysis and modification.* New York: Guilford.

Hahlweg, K., Revenstorf, D. & Schindler, L. (1984). Effects of behavioral marital therapy on couples' communication and problem solving skills. *Journal of Consulting and Clinical Psychology,* 52, 553–566.

Hansen, A., Hoogduin, C.A.L., Schaap, C. & deHaan, E. (1992). Do dropouts differ from successfully treated obsessive–compulsives? *Behavior Research and Therapy,* 30(5), 547–550.

Hartley, D.E. & Strupp, H.H. (1982). The therapeutic alliance: Its relationship to outcome in brief psychotherapy. In J. Masling (Ed.), *Empirical studies of psychoanalytical theories.* Hillsdale, NJ: Analytic Press.

Hattie, J.A., Sharpley, C.F., & Rogers, H.J. (1984). Comparative effectiveness of professional and paraprofessional helpers. *Psychological Bulletin,* 95, 534–541.

Heider, F. (1944). Social perception and phenomenal causality. *Psychological Review,* 51, 358–374.

Helner, P.A. & Jessel, J.C. (1974). Effects of interpretation as a counseling technique. *Journal of Counseling Psychology,* 21, 475–481.

Henrich, G. & Hahlweg, K. (1987). *On the pragmatics of sequential analysis: Comparing two frequently used methods in marital and family research.* Munich: Max Planck Institute for Psychiatry.

Henry, W.E., Sims, J.H. & Spray, S.L. (1971). *The fifth profession: Becoming a psychotherapist.* San Francisco: Jossey-Bass.

Henry, W.P., Schacht, T.E. & Strupp, H.H. (1986). Structural analysis of social behavior: Application to a study of interpersonal process in differential psychotherapeutic outcome. *Journal of Consulting and Clinical Psychology,* 34, 27–31.

Heppner, P.P. & Claiborn, C.D. (1989). Social influence research in counseling: A review and critique. *Journal of Counseling Psychology,* 36, 365–387.

Hewstone, M. (Ed.) (1983) *Attribution theory: Social and functional extensions.* Oxford: Blackwells.

Herschbach, P., Klinger, A. & Odefey, S. (1980). Die Therapeut-Klient Beziehung. Forschungsergebnisse und -perspektiven. Salzburg: Otto Müller.

Hill, C.E. (1978). Development of a counselor verbal response category system. *Journal of Counseling Psychology,* 25, 461–468.

Hill, C.E. (1982). Counseling process research: Philosophical and methodological dilemmas. *The Counseling Psychologist,* 30, 3–18.

Hill, C.E., Carter, J.A. & O'Farrell, M.K. (1983). A case study of the process and outcome of time-limited counseling. *Journal of Counseling Psychology,* 30, 3–18.

Hill, C.E. & Gormally, J. (1977). Effects of reflection, restatements, probe and nonverbal behaviors on client effect. *Journal of Counseling Psychology,* 24, 92–97.

Hill, C.E., Greenwald, C., Reed, K.G., Charles, D., O'Farrell, M.K. & Carter, J.A. (1981). *Manual for the counselor and client verbal response category system.* Columbus: Marathon.

Hill, C.E., Helms, J.E., Tichenor, V., Spiegel, S.B., O'Grady K.E. & Perry, E.S. (1988). Effects of therapist response modes in brief psychotherapy. *Journal of Counseling Psychotherapy,* 35, 222–233.

Hill, C.E., Thames, T.B. & Rardin, D.K. (1979). Comparison of Rogers, Pearls and Ellis on the Hill Counselor Verbal Response Category System. *Journal of Counseling Psychology*, 26, 198–203.

Hochdörfer, B., Ludwig, K., Rhenius, D. & Lasgoga, F. (1983). Zur Interaktion von Klient und Therapeut in der klientenzentrierten Gesprächstherapie. [On client–therapist interaction in client-centered verbal therapy] *Zeitschrift für Sozialpsychologie*, 14, 177–188.

Homans, G.L. (1961, 1974), *Social behavior: Its elementary forms*. New York: Harcourt Brace Jovanovich.

Hoogduin, C.A.L. & Duivenvoorden, H. (1988). A decision model in the treatment of obsessive–compulsive neurosis. *British Journal of Psychiatry*, 152, 516–521.

Hoogduin, C.A.L., Haan, E. de, & Schaap, C. (1989). The significance of the patient–therapist relationship in the treatment of obsessive-compulsive neurosis. *British Journal of Clinical Psychology*, 28, 185–186.

Hoogduin, C.A.L., Haan, E. de, Schaap, C., & Severeijns, R. (1988). De predicerende betekenis van de therapeutische relatie bij de behandeling van dwangneurose. [The predictive significance of the therapeutic relationship in the treatment of obsessive–compulsive neurosis] *Gedragstherapie*, 21(3), 247–257.

Hoorens, V. (1986). De cliënt–therapeut relatie in gedragstherapie. [The client–therapist relationship in behaviour therapy] *Gedragstherapie*, 19, 263–278.

Hopkinson, K., Cox, A. & Rutter, M. (1981). Psychiatric interviewing techniques. III. Naturalistic study: Eliciting feelings. *British Journal of Psychiatry*, 138, 406–415.

Jacobson, E. (1938). *Progressive relaxation*. Chicago: University of Chicago Press.

Janis, J.L. (1982). Helping relationships: A preliminary theoretical analysis. In I.L. Janis (Ed.), *Counseling on personal decisions: Theory and research on short-term helping relationship*. New Haven: Yale University Press.

Jessen, B. (1989). *Dropout bij ambulante psychotherapie*. [Dropout in outpatient psychotherapy] Master's Thesis, Department of Clinical Psychology and Personality, University of Nijmegen.

Jilek, W.G. (1974). *Salish Indians' mental health and cultural change*. Toronto: Holt.

Johnson, D.W. & Matross, R. (1977). Interpersonal influence in psychotherapy: A social psychology view. In A.S. Gurman & A.M. Razin (Eds.), *Effective psychotherapy*. New York: Pergamon.

Jourard, S.M. (1971). *Self-disclosure*. New York: Wiley.

Jourard, S.M. & Jaffé, P.E. (1970). Influence of an interviewer's self-disclosure on the self-disclosure behavior of interviewees. *Journal of Counseling Psychology*, 17, 252–257.

Kagan, N., Krathwohl, D.R. & Miller, R. (1963). Stimulated recall in therapy using videotape: A case study. *Journal of Counseling Psychology*, 10, 237–243.

Kaimer, P., Reinecker, H. & Schindler, L. (1989). Interaktionsmuster von Klient und Therapeut bei zwei unterschiedlich erfolgreich behandelten Fallen. [Interaction pattern of client and therapist in two distinct successful cases] *Zeitschrift für Klinische Psychologie*, 28, 80–92.

Kanfer, F.H. (1984). Self-management in clinical and social interventions. In R.P. McGlynn, J.E. Maddux, C.D. Stoltenberg & J.H. Harvey, (Eds.), *Social perception in clinical and counseling psychology*. Lubbock, TX: Texas Press.

Kanfer, F.H. & Grimm, L.G. (1980). Managing clinical change: A process model of therapy. *Behavior Modification*, 4, 419–444.

Kanfer, F.H., Philips, J.S., Matarazzo, J.D. & Saslow, G. (1960). Experimental modification of interviewer content in standardized interviews. *Journal of Counseling Psychology*, 24, 528–536.

Kanfer, F.H. & Philips, J.S. (1970). *Learning foundations of behavior therapy*. New York: Wiley.

178 References

Kanfer, F.H., Reinecker, H. & Schmelzer, D. (1990). *Selbstmanagement- Therapie als Veranderungsprocess: Ein Lehrbuch für die Klinische Praxis.* [Self-management therapy as change process] Heidelberg: Springer.

Kanfer, F.H. & Saslow, G. (1974). Verhaltenstheoretische Diagnostik. [Behaviour theoretical diagnostics] In D. Schulte (Ed.), *Diagnostik in der Verhaltenstherapie.* [Diagnostics in behaviour therapy] München: Urban & Schwarzenberg.

Kanfer, F.H. & Schefft, B.K. (1988). *Guiding the process of therapeutic change.* Campaign: Research Press.

Kaschak, E. (1978). Therapist and client: Two views of the process and outcome of psychotherapy. *Professional Psychology,* 9, 271-277.

Kazdin, A.E. (1979). Fictions, factions and functions of behavior therapy. *Behavior Therapy,* 10, 629-654.

Kazdin, A.E. (1986). Research designs and methodology. In S.L. Garfield & A.E. Bergin (Eds.), *Handbook of psychotherapy and behavior change.* New York: Wiley.

Kazdin, A.E. & Wilcoxon, L.A. (1976). Systematic desensitization and nonspecific treatment effects: A methodological evaluation. *Psychological Bulletin,* 83, 729-758.

Keijsers, G.P.J., Schaap, C. & Hoogduin, C.A.L. (1990). Therapeutic relationship enhancement procedures and the Social Power Model. In H.G. Zapotoczky & T. Wenzel (Eds.), *The scientific dialogue: From basic research to clinical intervention.* Lisse/Amsterdam: Swets & Zeitlinger.

Keijsers, G.P.J., Schaap, C. & Hoogduin, C.A.L. (1992) *De Therapist Client Rating Scale (TCRS): Meer data over de structuur en validiteit* [The Therapist–Client Rating Scale (TCRS): More data on the structure and validity.] *Gedragstherapie,* 25, 201-210.

Keijsers, G.P.J., Schaap, C., Hoogduin, C.A.L. & Peters, W. (1991). The therapeutic relationship in the behavioural treatment of anxiety disorders. *Behavioural Psychotherapy,* 19, 359-367.

Keijsers, L.H.A., Schaap, C., Keijsers, G.P.J., & Hoogduin, C.A.L. (1990). Interactiestijl, psychotherapie en persoonlijkheidsstoornis. [Interaction style, psychotherapy and personality disorder] In C. van der Staak & C. Hoogduin (Eds.), *Diagnostiek en behandeling van de persoonlijkheidsstoornis.* [Diagnostics and treatment of personality disorder] Nijmegen: Bureau Beta.

Keithley, L.J. (1985). Patient motivation: Its relation to improvement in psychotherapy, premature termination and therapist attitudes and behavior. *Dissertation Abstracts International,* 45(12-B), 3946.

Kelley, H.H. & Thibaut, J.W. (1978). *Interpersonal relations: A theory of interdependence.* New York: Wiley.

Kernberg, O.F., Burnstein, E.D., Cayle, L., Appelbaum, A., Horwitz, L. & Vath, H. (1972). Psychotherapy and psychoanalysis: Final report of the Menninger Foundation's Psychotherapy Research Project. *Bulletin of the Menninger Clinic,* 36, 1-276.

Kersten, T. (1987). *De (tegen)werking van weerstand.* [The (counter)productivity of resistance] Master's Thesis, University of Nijmegen.

Kersten, T., Hoogduin, C.A.L. & Schaap, C. (1988). *Instrumenten om motivatie voor psychotherapie te meten: Een overzicht.* [Instruments to measure motivation for psychotherapy: A review] Internal Report. University of Nijmegen, Department of Clinical Psychology and Personality.

Keupp, H. (1979). Die Kontroverse um das richtige Verständnis von psychischer Störung und Normalität. [The controversy regarding the right understanding of psychiatric disturbance and normality] In H. Keupp (Hrsg.), *Normalität und Abweichung.* [Normality and deviance] Munich: Urban & Schwarzenberg.

Kiesler, D.J. (1971). Experimental designs in psychotherapy research. In A.E. Bergin & S.L. Garfield (Eds.), *Handbook of psychotherapy and behavior change*. New York: Wiley.

Kiesler, D.J. (1979). An interpersonal communication analysis of relationship in psychotherapy. *Psychiatry*, 24, 299–311.

Kiesler, D.J. (1982). Confronting the client–therapist relationship in psychotherapy. In J.C. Anchin & D.J. Kiesler (Eds.), *Handbook of interpersonal psychotherapy*. New York: Pergamon.

Kiesler, D.J. (1983). The interpersonal circle: a taxonomy for the complementarity in human transactions. *Psychological Review*, 90, 185–214.

Kiesler, D.J., Mathieu, P.L. & Klein, M.H. (1965). Sampling from recorded therapy interview: The problem of segment location. *Journal of Consulting Psychology*, 29, 337–344.

Klein, M.H., Mathieu, P.L., Gendlin, E.T. & Kiesler, D.J. (1969). *The experiencing scale*. Madison, WI: Wisconsin Psychiatric Institute.

Knapp, M.L. (1978). *Social intercourse: From greeting to goodbye*. Boston: Allyn and Bacon.

Krasner, L. (1962). The therapist as a social reinforcement machine. In H.H. Strupp & L. Luborsky (Eds.), *Research in psychotherapy*. Washington, DC: APA.

Krause, M.S. (1964). Twelve propositions in the semantics of motivation. *The Journal of General Psychology*, 70, 331–339.

Krause, M.S. (1966). A cognitive theory of motivation for treatment. *Journal of General Psychology*, 75, 9–19.

Krause, M.S. (1967). Behavioral indexes of motivation for treatment. *Journal of Counseling Psychology*, 14, 426–435.

Krause, M.S. (1968). Clarification at intake and motivation for treatment. *Journal of Counseling Psychology*, 15, 576–577.

Krippner, S. (1975). *Song of the siren: A parapsychological odyssey*. New York: Harper.

Labov, W. & Fanshel, D. (1977). *Therapeutic discourse: Psychotherapy as conversation*. New York: Academic Press.

Lambert, M.J. & Ayas, T.P. (1984). Patient characteristics and their relationship to psychotherapy outcome. In M. Hersen, L. Michelson & A.S. Bellack (Eds.), *Issues in psychotherapy research*. New York: Plenum.

Lambert, M.J., De Julio, S.S. & Stein, D.M. (1978). Therapist interpersonal skills: Process, outcome, methodological considerations and recommendations for future research. *Psychological Bulletin*, 85, 467–489.

Lange, A. (1987). *Strategieën in directieve therapie*. [Strategies in directive therapy] Deventer: Van Loghum Slaterus.

Lavalle, J.J. (1977). Comparing the effects of an affective and a behavioral counselor style on client interview behavior. *Journal of Counseling Psychology*, 24, 173–177.

Lazarus, A.A. (1958). New methods in psychotherapy: A case study. *South African Medical Journal*, 32, 660–664.

Leary, T. (1957). *Interpersonal diagnosis of personality*. New York: Donald.

Lee, D.Y., Hallberg, E.T. & Harrard, J.H. (1979). Client verbal and non-verbal reinforcement of counselor behavior: Its impact on interviewing behavior and postinterview evaluation. *Journal of Counseling Psychology*, 16, 204–209.

Lee, D.Y. & Uhleman, M.R. (1984). Comparison of verbal responses of Rogers, Shostrom and Lazarus. *Journal of Counseling Psychology*, 31, 91–94.

Leitenberg, N., Agras, W.S., Allen, R., Butz, R. & Edwards, J. (1975). Feedback and therapist praise during treatment of a phobia. *Journal of Consulting and Clinical Psychology*, 43, 396–404.

Lenihan, G.O., Sanders, C.D. (1984). Guidelines for group therapy with eating disorders victims. *Journal of Counseling and Development*, 63, 252–254.

Lick, J. & Bootzin, R. (1975). Expectancy factors in the treatment of fear: Methodological and theoretical issues. *Psychological Bulletin*, 82, 917–931.

Lietaer, G. (1976). Nederlandstalige revisie van Barrett-Lennard's Relationship Inventory voor individueel-therapeutische relaties. [Dutch revision of Barrett-Lennard's Relationship Inventory for individual therapeutic relationships] *Psychologica Belgica*, 16, 73–94.

Llewelyn, S.P. & Hume, W.I. (1979). The patient's view of therapy. *British Journal of Medical Psychology*, 52, 29–35.

Locke, E.A. (1971). Is "behavior therapy" behavioristic? An analysis of Wolpe's psychotherapeutic methods. *Psychological Bulletin*, 76, 318–327.

Lorr, M. (1965). Client perceptions of therapists: A study of the therapeutic relation. *Journal of Consulting Psychology*, 29, 146–149.

Lorr, M. & McNair, D.M. (1965). Expansion of the Interpersonal Behavior Circle. *Journal of Personality and Social Psychology*, 2, 823–830.

Luborsky, L. (1976). Helping alliances in psychotherapy. In J.L. Claghorn (Ed.), *Successful Psychotherapy*. New York: Brunner/Mazel.

Luborsky, L. (1984). *Principles of psychoanalytic psychotherapy: A manual for supportive–expressive treatment*. New York: Basic Books.

Luborsky, L., Mintz, J., Auerbach, A., Christoph, P., Bachrach, H., Todd, T., Johnson, M., Cohen, M. & O'Brien, C.P. (1980). Predicting the outcome of psychotherapy. *Archives of General Psychiatry*, 37, 471.

Lutz, R. (1978). *Das verhaltensdiagnostische Interview*. [The behaviour-diagnostic interview] Stuttgart: Kohlhammer.

Maddux, J.E., Stoltenberg, C.D. & Rosenwein, R. (Eds.) (1987). *Social processes in clinical and counseling psychology*. New York: Springer.

Mahoney, M.J. (1974). *Cognition and behavior modification*. Cambridge: Ballinger.

Mahrer, A.R., Nifakis, D.J., Abhukara, L. & Sterner, I. (1984). Microstrategies in psychotherapy: The patterning of sequential therapist statements. *Psychotherapy*, 21, 465–472.

Major, B. & Haslin, R. (1982). Perceptions of cross-sex and same-sex nonreciprocal touch: It's better to give than to receive. *Journal of Nonverbal Behavior*, 6, 148–162.

Mann, B. & Murphy, K.C. (1975). Timing of self-disclosure, reciprocity of self-disclosure and reactions to an initial interview. *Journal of Counseling Psychology*, 22, 304–308.

Margolin, G. & Wampold, B.E. (1981). Sequential analysis of conflict and accord in distressed and non-distressed marital partners. *Journal of Consulting and Clinical Psychology*, 49, 554–567.

Marks, I.M. (1987). *Fears, phobias and rituals*. Oxford: Oxford University Press.

Marsden, G. (1965). Content-analysis studies of therapeutic interviews: 1954–1964. *Psychological Bulletin*, 63, 298–321.

Marston, A.R. (1984). What makes therapists run? Model for analysis of motivation styles. *Psychotherapy*, 21, 456–459.

Martin, D.G. (1971). *Learning-based client-centered therapy*. Belmont: Brooks/Cole.

Marziali, E. (1984). Three viewpoints on the therapeutic alliance. *The Journal of Nervous and Mental Disease*, 172, 417–423.

Marziali, E., Marmar, C. & Krupnick, J. (1981). Therapeutic alliance scales: Development and relationship to psychotherapy outcome. *American Journal of Psychiatry*, 138, 361–364.

McCormack, M.H. (1984). *What they don't teach you at Harvard Business School*. Glasgow: Fontana.

McDaniel, S.H., Stiles, W.B. & McGaughey, K.J. (1981). Correlations of male college student's verbal response mode use in psychotherapy with measures of psychological disturbance and psychotherapy outcome. *Journal of Consulting and Clinical Psychology*, 49, 571–582.

McGlynn, F.D. (1976). Comment on the Morris and Suckerman study of therapist warmth as a factor in automated systematic desensitization. *Journal of Consulting and Clinical Psychology*, 44, 483–489.

McGuire, W.J. (1985). Attitudes and attitude change. In G. Lindsey & E. Aronson. *Handbook of Social Psychology* (Vol. 2), *Special fields and applications*, 3rd Edition. New York: Newberry Award Records.

McNair, D., Lorr, M. & Callahan, D. (1963). Patient and therapist influences on quitting therapy. *Journal of Consulting Psychology*, 27, 10–17.

McNeill, B.W. & Stoltenberg, C.D. (1989). Reconceptualizing social influence in counseling: The elaboration likelihood model. *Journal of Counseling Psychology*, 36, 24–33.

Meara, N.M., Shannon, J.W. & Pepinsky, H.B. (1979). Comparison of the stylistic complexity of the language of counselor and client across three theoretical orientations. *Journal of Counseling Psychology*, 26, 181–189.

Meichenbaum, D. (1971). Examination of model characteristics in reducing avoidance behavior. *Journal of Personality and Social Psychology*, 14, 298–307.

Meier, A. & Boivin, M. (1986). Client verbal response category system: Preliminary data. *Journal of Consulting and Clinical Psychology*, 54, 877–879.

Miller, W.R. (1985). Motivation for treatment: A review with special emphasis on alcoholism. *Psychological Bulletin*, 98, 1, 84–107.

Millon, T. (1981). *Disorders of personality: DSM-III Axis II*. New York: Wiley.

Mintz, J., Auerbach, A.H., Luborsky, L. & Johnson, M. (1973). Patient's, therapist's and observers' views of psychotherapy: A "Rashomon" experience or a reasonable consensus? *British Journal of Medical Psychology*, 46, 83–89.

Mintz, J. & Luborsky, L. (1971). Segments vs. whole session: Which is better unit for psychotherapy process research? *Journal of Abnormal Psychology*, 78, 180–191.

Mintz, J., Luborsky, L. & Auerbach, A.H. (1971). Dimensions of psychotherapy: A factor-analytic study of ratings of psychotherapy sessions. *Journal of Consulting and Clinical Psychology*, 36, 106–120.

Morris, R.J. & Suckerman, K.R. (1974). Therapist warmth as a factor in automated systematic desensitization. *Journal of Consulting and Clinical Psychology*, 42, 244–250.

Murphy, P.M., Cramer, D. & Lillie, F.J. (1984). The relationship between curative factors perceived by patients in their psychotherapy and treatment outcome: An exploratory study. *British Journal of Medical Psychology*, 57, 187–192.

Nawas, M.M., Pluk, P.W. & Wojciechowski, F.L. (1985). In search of the nonspecific factors in psychotherapy: A speculative essay. In M.A. v. Kalmthout, C. Schaap & F.L. Wojciechowski (Eds.), *Common factors in psychotherapy*. Lisse: Swets & Zeitlinger.

O'Dell, S.L. (1982). Enhancing parent involvement training: A discussion. *The Behavior Therapist*, 5, 9–13.

O'Dell, J.W. & Bahmer, A.J. (1981). Rogers, Lazarus and Shostrom in content analysis. *Journal of Clinical Psychology*, 37, 507.

O'Malley, S.S., Suh, C.S. & Strupp, H.H. (1983). The Vanderbilt Psychotherapy Process Scale: A report on the scale development and a process-outcome study. *Journal of Consulting and Clinical Psychology*, 51, 581–586.

Orlinsky, D.E. & Howard, K.I. (1966). *Therapy session report, forms P and T*. Chicago: Institute for Juvenile Research.

Orlinsky, D.E. & Howard, K.I. (1975). *Varieties of psychotherapeutic experience.* New York: Teacher's College.

Orlinsky, D.E. & Howard, K.I. (1978). The relation of process to outcome in psychotherapy. In S.L. Garfield & A.E. Bergin (Eds.), *Handbook of psychotherapy and behavior change.* New York: Wiley.

Orlinsky, D.E. & Howard, K.I. (1986). The psychological interior of psychotherapy: Explorations with the therapy session reports. In L.S. Greenberg & W.M. Pinsof (Eds.), *The psychotherapeutic process. A research handbook.* New York: Guilford.

Osgood, C.E., May, W. & Miron, M. (1975). *Cross-cultural universals of affective meaning.* Urbana: University of Illinois Press.

Parloff, M.B., Waskow, I.E. & Wolfe, B.E. (1978). Research on therapist variables in relation to process and outcome. In S.C. Garfield & A.E. Bergin (Eds.), *Handbook of psychotherapy and behavior change.* New York: Wiley.

Patterson, C.H. (1968). Relationship therapy and/or behavior therapy. *Psychotherapy,* **5,** 226–233.

Patterson, G.R. (1976). The agressive child: Victim and architect of a coercive system. In A. Hamerlynck, F. Handy & V. Mash (Eds.), *Behavior Modification and Families: I. Theory and Research.* New York; Brunner/Mazel.

Patterson, G.R. (1982). *A social learning approach: Coercive family process.* Eugene OR: Castalia.

Pekarik, G. (1983). Improvement in clients who have given different reasons for dropping out of treatment. *Journal of Counseling Psychology,* **39,** 909–913.

Perkins, J., Kiesler, D.J., Anchin, J.C., Chirico, B.M., Kyle, E.M. & Federman, E.J. (1979). The Impact Message Inventory: A new measure of relationship in counseling/psychotherapy and other dyads. *Journal of Counseling Psychology,* **35,** 363–367.

Phillips, E. (1985). *Psychotherapy Revised: New frontiers in research and practice.* Hillsdale: Earlbaum.

Pope, B. (1979). *The mental health interview: Research and application.* New York: Pergamon.

Pope, B., Blass, T., Siegman, A.W. & Raher, J. (1970). Anxiety and depression in speech. *Journal of Consulting and Clinical Psychology,* **35,** 128–133.

Powell, N.J. (1968). Differential effectiveness of interviewer interventions in an experimental interview. *Journal of Consulting and Clinical Psychology,* **32,** 210–215.

Prioleau, L., Murdock, M. & Brody, N. (1983). An analysis of psychotherapy versus placebo studies. *The Behavioral and Brain Sciences,* **2,** 275–285.

Prince, R.H. (1964). Indigenous Yoruba psychiatry. In A. Kiev (Ed.), *Magic, faith and healing.* New York: Free Press.

Proctor, E.K. & Rosen, A. (1983). Structure in therapy: A conceptual analysis. *Psychotherapy,* **20,** 202–207.

Rabavilas, A.D., Boulougouris, I.C. & Perissaki, C. (1979). Therapist qualities related to outcome with exposure in vivo in neurotic patients. *Journal of Behavior Therapy and Experimental Psychiatry,* **10,** 293–294.

Reid, W.J. & Shapiro, B.L. (1969). Client reactions to advice. *The Social Service Review,* **43,** 165–173.

Reinecker, H. (1986). Grundlagen verhaltenstherapeutischer Methoden. [Foundations of behaviour therapeutic methods] In: DGVT (Ed.), *Verhaltenstherapie: Theorien und Methoden.* [Behaviour therapy: Theories and methods] Tübingen: DGVT.

Reinecker, H. (1987). *Grundlagen der Verhaltenstherapie.* [Foundations of behaviour therapy] München: Psychologie Verlags Union.

Revenstorf, D., Hahlweg, K., Schindler, L. & Vogel, B. (1984). Interaction analysis of marital conflict. In K. Hahlweg & N. Jacobson (Eds.), *Marital interaction: Analysis and modification.* New York: Guilford.

Rice, L.N. (1965). Therapist's style of participation and cause outcome. *Journal of Consulting Psychology*, **29**, 155–160.

Rice, L.N. (1983). The relationship in client-centered therapy. In M.J. Lambert (Ed.), *A guide to psychotherapy and patient relationship*. Homewood: Dow Jones-Irwin.

Rice, L.N. & Greenberg, L.S. (Eds.) (1984). *Patterns of change: Intensive analysis of psychotherapy process*. New York: Guilford.

Rice, L.N. & Wagstaff, A.K. (1967). Client voice quality and expressive style as indexes of productive psychotherapy. *Journal of Consulting Psychology*, **31**, 557–563.

Ringler, M. (1977). Der Einfluss von demokratischem vs. autoritärem Therapeutenverhalten auf Erfolg, Erfolgserwartung und Self-Attribution bei Desensibilisierung von Prüfungsangst. [The effect of democratic versus authoritarian therapist behaviour on success, success-expectation and self-attribution in desensitization of examination anxiety] *Zeitschrift für Klinische Psychologie*, **6**, 40–58.

Rogers, W.T. & Jones, S.E. (1975). Effects of dominance tendencies in floor holding and interruption behavior in dyadic interaction. *Human Communication Research*, **1**, 113–122.

Rosenbaum, R.L. & Horowitz, M.J. (1983). Motivation for psychotherapy: A factorial and conceptual analysis. *Psychotherapy*, **20**, 346–354.

Rosenthal, D. & Frank, J.D. (1956). Psychotherapy and the placebo effect. *Psychological Bulletin*, **53**, 294–302.

Rosenthal, T.L. (1980). Social cueing processes. In M. Hersen, R.M. Eisler & I.M. Miller (Eds.), *Progress in behavior modification*. New York: Academic Press.

Russell, R.C. & Stiles, W.B. (1979). Categories for classifying language in psychotherapy. *Psychological Bulletin*, **86**, 404–419.

Russell, R.C. & Trull, T.J. (1986). Sequential analysis of language variables in psychotherapy process research. *Journal of Consulting and Clinical Psychology*, **54**, 16–21.

Ryan, V.L. & Gyzynski, M.N. (1971). Behaviour therapy in retrospect: Patients' feelings about their behaviour therapies. *Journal of Consulting and Clinical Psychology*, **37**, 1–9.

Sackett, G. (1978). The lag sequential analysis of contingency and cyclicity in behavioral interaction research. In J. Osofsky (Ed.), *Handbook of infant development*. New York: Wiley.

Saltzman, M.J., Luetgert, M.J., Roth, J.C. & Howard, L. (1976). Formation of a therapeutic relationship: Experiences during the initial phase of psychotherapy as predictors of treatment duration and outcome. *Journal of Consulting and Clinical Psychology*, **44**, 546–555.

Schaap, C. (1982). *Communication and adjustment in marriage*. Lisse: Swets & Zeitlinger.

Schaap, C. (1984). A comparison of the interaction of distressed and nondistressed couples in a laboratory situation: Literature review, methodological issues, and an empirical investigation. In K. Hahlweg & N.S. Jacobson (Eds.), *Marital interaction: Analysis and modification*. New York: Guilford.

Schaap, C., Buunk, A., & Kerkstra, A. (1988). Marital conflict resolution. In P. Noller, & M.A. Fitzpatrick (Eds.), *Perspectives in marital interaction*. Clevedon, UK: Multilingual Matters Ltd.

Schaap. C., & Hoogduin, C. (1988). The therapeutic relationship in behaviour therapy: Enhancing the quality of the bond. In P.G.M. Emmelkamp (Ed.), *Advances in theory and practice in behaviour therapy*. Lisse: Swets & Zeitlinger.

Schaap, C., Hoogduin, C.A.L., Keijsers, G., & Kersten, T. (1989). Motiveringstechnieken als processen van sociale beïnvloeding. [Motivation techniques as processes of social influence] In A.P. Buunk, & A. Vrugt (Eds.), *Sociale psychologie en psychische problemen: Op het raakvlak van sociale en klinische psychologie.* [Social psychology and psychiatric problems: On the interface between social and clinical psychology] Assen, The Netherlands: Dekker van de Vegt.

Schaap, C., & Jansen-Nawas, C. (1987). Marital interaction, affect and conflict resolution. *Sexual and Marital Therapy,* **2,** 12–24.

Schaap, C. & Schippers, G.M. (1986). Motivation strategies in the behavioral treatment of problem drinkers. XVIth Annual Conference of the European Association for Behaviour Therapy, Lausanne, Switzerland, September.

Schaap, C. & Suntjes, H. (1986). *Therapeutic style in psychotherapy and behaviour therapy.* XVIth Annual Conference of the EABT, Lausanne, Switzerland, Sept 1986.

Schaffer, N.D. (1982). Multidimensional measures of therapist behavior as predictors of outcome. *Psychological Bulletin,* **92,** 670–681.

Scherer, K.R. (1979). Voice and speech correlates of perceived social influences in simulated juries. In H. Giles & R. St. Clair (Eds.), *Language and social behavior.* Baltimore MD: University Park Press.

Schindler, L. (1988). Client–therapist interaction and therapeutic change. In P. Emmelkamp, W. Everaerd, F. Kraaimaat & M. van Son (Eds.), *Advances in theory and practice in behaviour therapy.* Lisse: Swets & Zeitlinger.

Schindler, L. (1990). Schlafstorungen. [Sleep disturbances] In Reinecker, H. (Ed.), *Lehrbuch der Klinische Psychologie.* [Handbook of clinical psychology] Göttingen: Hogrefe.

Schindler, L., Hohenberger-Sieber, E. & Hahlweg, K. (1989). Observing client–therapist interaction in behaviour therapy: Development and first application of an observational system. *British Journal of Clinical Psychology,* **28,** 213–226.

Schindler, L. Müller, U., Hohenberger-Sieber, E. & Hahlweg, K. (1988). *Codiersystem zur Interaktion in der Psychotherapie (CIP): Manual für den Beobachter.* [Coding system for interaction in psychotherapy (CIP): Manual for the observer] Munich: Max Planck Institute for Psychiatry.

Schindler, L., Revenstorf, D., Hahlweg, K. & Brengelman, J.C. (1983). Therapeutenverhalten in der Verhaltenstherapie: Entwicklung eines Instruments zur Beurteilung durch den Klienten. [Therapist behaviour in behaviour therapy: Development of an instrument for rating by the client] *Partnerberatung,* **20,** 149–157.

Schulte, D. (Ed.) (1974). *Diagnostik in der Verhaltenstherapie.* [Diagnostics in behaviour therapy] München: Urban & Schwarzenberg.

Schwab, R. & Mathiesen, C. (1979). Klienten-Selbstexploration und Helfermerkmale in quasi-therapeutischen einmaligen Gesprächen. [Client self-exploration and helper characteristics in quasi-therapeutic single sessions] *Zeitschrift für klinische Psychologie,* **8,** 204–212.

Schwab, R. & Tonnies, S. (1984). Klientenzentrierte Einzelpsychotherapie und personenzentrierte Gesprächsgruppen: Neuere Forschungsergebnisse und Entwicklungen. [Client-centered individual psychotherapy and person-centered group therapy: New outcome from research and developments] In U. Baumann, H. Berback & G. Seidenstöcker (Eds.), *Klinische Psychologie: Trends in Forschung und Praxis.* [Clinical psychology: Trends in research and practice] Bern: Huber.

Searle, J.R. (1969), *Speech acts: An essay in the philosophy of language.* Cambridge: Cambridge University Press.

Seltzer, L.F. (1986). *Paradoxical strategies in psychotherapy: A comprehensive review and guidebook.* New York: Wiley.

Shapiro, K. (1986). The placebo effect in medical and psychological therapies. In S.L. Garfield & A.E. Bergin (Eds.), *Handbook of psychotherapy and behavior change.* New York: Wiley.

Shapiro, D.A. & Shapiro, D. (1982). Meta-analysis of comparative therapy outcome studies: A replication and refinement. *Psychological Bulletin,* **92,** 581–604.

Shapiro, D.A., Barkham, M. & Irving, D.L. (1984). The reliability of modified helper behavior rating system. *British Journal of Medical Psychology*, 57, 45–48.

Shaw, M.E. (1981). *Group dynamics: The psychology of small group behavior.* New York: McGraw Hill.

Shoham-Salomon, U. & Rosenthal, R. (1987). Paradoxical Interventions: A meta-analysis. *Journal of Consulting and Clinical Psychology*, 55, 22–28.

Shostrom, E.L. (1966). *Three approaches to psychotherapy.* Santa Ana, CA: Psychological Films.

Shostrom, E.L. (1977). *Three approaches to psychotherapy II.* Santa Ana, CA: Psychological Films.

Shostrom, E.L. & Riley, C.M. (1968). Parametric analysis of psychotherapy. *Journal of Consulting and Clinical Psychology*, 32, 628-632.

Siegel, N. & Fink, M. (1962). Motivation for psychotherapy. *Comprehensive Psychiatry*, 3, 170–173.

Sifneos, P.E. (1971). Change in patients motivation for psychotherapy. *American Journal of Psychiatry*, 128, 718–721.

Sifneos, P.E. (1975). Criteria for psychotherapeutic outcome. *Psychotherapy and Psychosomatics*, 26, 49–58.

Silberschatz, G., Fretter, P.B. & Curtis, J.T. (1986). How do interpretations influence the process of psychotherapy? *Journal of Consulting and Clinical Psychology*, 54, 646–652.

Singer, B. & Luborsky, L. (1977). Countertransference: The status of clinical and quantitative research. In A.S. Gurman & A.M. Razin (Eds.), *Effective psychotherapy.* New York: Pergamon.

Sloane, R.B., Staples, F.R., Cristol, A.H., Yorkston, N.J. & Whipple, K. (1975). *Psychotherapy versus behavior therapy.* Cambridge, MA: Harvard University Press.

Sloane, R.B., Staples, F.R., Whipple, K. & Cristol, A.H. (1977). Patients' attitudes toward behavior therapy and psychotherapy. *American Journal of Psychiatry*, 134, 134–137.

Smith, M.L., Glass, G.V. & Miller, T.I. (1980). *The benefits of psychotherapy.* Baltimore, MD: Johns Hopkins University Press.

Snyder, W.U. (1945). An investigation of the nature of nondirective psychotherapy. *The Journal of General Psychology*, 33, 193–223.

Spielberger, L.D. & DeNike, L.D. (1966). Descriptive behaviorism versus cognitive theory in verbal operant conditioning. *Psychological Review*, 73, 306–326.

Staples, F.R., Sloane, R.B., Whipple, K., Cristol, A.H. & Yorkston, N.T. (1975). Differences between behavior therapists and psychotherapists. *Archives of General Psychiatry*, 32, 1517–1522.

Stiles, W.B. (1978). *Manual for taxonomy of verbal response modes.* Chapel Hill, NC: University of North Carolina Press.

Stiles, W.B. (1979). Verbal response modes and psychotherapeutic technique. *Psychiatry*, 42, 49–62.

Stiles, W.B. (1980). Measurement of the impact of psychotherapy sessions. *Journal of Consulting and Clinical Psychology*, 48, 176–185.

Stiles, W.B. (1986). Levels of intended meaning of utterances. *British Journal of Clinical Psychology*, 25, 213–222.

Stiles, W.B., McDaniel, S.H. & McGaughey, K. (1979). Verbal response mode correlates of experiencing. *Journal of Consulting and Clinical Psychology*, 47, 795–797.

Stiles, W.B. & Snow, J.S. (1984). Counseling session impact as viewed by novice counselors and their clients. *Journal of Counseling Psychology*, 31, 3–12.

Stiles, W.B. & Sultan, F.E. (1979). Verbal response mode use by clients in psychotherapy. *Journal of Consulting and Clinical Psychology*, 47, 611–613.

Street, R.L. Jr. & Hopper, R. (1982). A model of speech style evaluation. In E.B. Ryan & H. Giles (Eds.), *Attitudes towards language variation: Social and applied contexts*. London: Edward Arnold.

Strong, S.R. (1968). Counseling: An interpersonal influence process. *Journal of Counseling Psychology*, 15, 215–224.

Strong, S.R. (1978). Social psychology approach to psychotherapy research. In S. Garfield & A.E. Bergin (Eds.), *Handbook of psychotherapy and behavior change*. New York: Wiley.

Strong, S.R. (1982). Emerging integration of clinical and social psychology: A clinicians perspective. In G. Weary & H.L. Mirels (Eds.), *Integrations of clinical and social psychology*. New York: Oxford University Press.

Strong, S.R. & Claiborn, C.D. (1982). *Change through interaction*. New York: Wiley.

Strong, S.R. & Matross, R.P. (1973). Change processes in counseling and psychotherapy. *Journal of Counseling Psychology*, 20, 25–37.

Strong, S.R., Wambach, C.A., Lopez, F.G. & Cooper, R.K. (1979). Motivational and equipping functions of interpretation in counseling. *Journal of Counseling Psychology*, 26, 98–107.

Strupp, H.H. (1955). Psychotherapeutic technique, professional affiliation and experience level. *Journal of Consulting Psychology*, 19, 97–102.

Strupp, H.H. (1978). Psychotherapy research and practice: An overview. In S.L. Garfield & A.E. Bergin (Eds.), *Handbook of psychotherapy and behavior change: An empirical analysis*. New York: Wiley.

Strupp, H.H. & Hadley, S.W. (1979). Specific vs. nonspecific factors in psychotherapy. *Archives of General Psychiatry*, 36, 1125.

Strupp, H.H., Walach, M.S. & Wogan, M. (1964). Psychotherapy experience in retrospect: Questionnaire survey of former patients and their therapists. *Psychological Monographs*, 78.

Suh, C.S., Strupp, H.H. & O'Malley, S.S. (1986). The Vanderbilt Process Measures: The Psychotherapy Process Scale and the Negative Indicators Scale. In L.S. Greenberg & W.M. Pinsof (Eds.), *The psychotherapeutic process: A research handbook*. New York: Guilford.

Sullivan, H.S. (1953). *Interpersonal theory of personality*. New York: Norton.

Swan, G.E. & McDonald, M.L. (1978). Behavior therapy in practice: A national survey of behavior therapists. *Behavior Therapy*, 9, 799–807.

Sweet, A.A. (1984). The therapeutic relationship in behavior therapy. *Clinical Psychology Review*, 4, 253–272.

Tennen, H., Rohrbach, M., Press, S. & White, L. (1981). Reactance theory and therapeutic paradox: A compliance-defiance model. *Psychotherapy*, 18, 14–21.

Thibaut, J. & Kelley, H.H. (1959). *The social psychology of groups*. New York: Wiley.

Torrey, E.F. (1972). What Western psychotherapists can learn from witchdoctors. *American Journal of Orthopsychiatry*, 42, 69–76.

Tracey, T.J. (1986). Interactional correlates of premature termination. *Journal of Consulting and Clinical Psychology*, 54, 784–788.

Truax, C.B. (1970). Therapist's evaluative statements and patient outcome in psychotherapy. *Journal of Clinical Psychology*, 26, 536–538.

Truax, C.B. & Carkhuff, R.R. (1967). *Toward effective counseling and psychotherapy*. Chicago: Aldine.

Truax, C.B. & Wittmer, J. (1971). Patient non-personal reference during psychotherapy and therapeutic outcome. *Journal of Clinical Psychology*, 27, 300–302.

Turkat, J.D. (1986). The behavioral interview. In A.R. Ciminero, K.S. Calhoun & H.E. Adams (Eds.). *Handbook of behavioral assessment*. New York: Wiley.

Vahia, N.S. (1973). Psychophysiological therapy based on the concept of Tatanjali. *American Journal of Psychotherapy*, 27, 557–565.

Van Bohemen, T. (1987). *Het meten van weerstandsgedrag in psychotherapie.* [Measuring resistant behaviour in psychotherapy] Master's Thesis, University of Nijmegen.

Van der Velden, K. (1985). Eclecticisme als noodsprong: Mededelingen uit het 'moeilijke mensen' project. [Eclecticism as an emergency jump: Communications from the "difficult people" project] *Kwartaalschrift voor Directieve Therapie en Hypnose*, 5, 393–410.

Van der Velden, K. & Van Dyck, R. (1977). Motiveringstechnieken. [Motivation techniques] In K. van der Velden (Ed.), *Directieve therapie Deel I.* [Directive therapy Part I] Deventer: Van Loghum Slaterus.

Van Dijk, P. (1979). *Geneeswijzen in Nederland.* [Healing methods in the Netherlands] Deventer: Ankh-Hermes.

Van Dyck, R. (1986). *Psychotherapie, placebo en suggestie* [Psychotherapy, placebo and suggestion] Doctoral Dissertation, University of Leiden, The Netherlands.

Van Dyck, R. & Emmelkamp, P. (1985). Eclecticisme: Een stap in de goede richting? [Eclecticism: A step in the right direction?] *Kwartaalschrift voor Directieve Therapie en Hypnose*, 5, 303–318.

Van Dyck, R., Van der Velden, K. & Emmelkamp, P. (1991). Algemene therapiefactoren, eclecticisme en indicatiestelling voor psychotherapie. In W. Vandereycken, C. Hoogduin, & P. Emmelkamp (Eds.), *Handboek Psychopathologie: Deel 2.* Houten/Antwerpen: Bohn Stafleu Van Loghum.

Van Kalmthout, M., Schaap, C. & Wojciechowski, F.L. (Eds.) (1985). *Common factors in psychotherapy.* Lisse: Swets & Zeitlinger.

Walrond-Skinner, S. (1986). *A dictionary of psychotherapy.* New York: Routledge and Kegan Paul.

Wampold, B.E. & Margolin, G.A. (1982). Nonparametric strategies to test the independence of behavioral states in sequential data. *Psychological Bulletin*, 92, 755–765.

Watzlawick, P., Beavin, J. & Jackson, D. (1967). *Pragmatics of human communication.* New York: Norton.

Weber, R.L. (1984). Antecedents of clinician judgement concerning patient motivation. *Dissertation Abstracts International*, 45(3-B), 1034.

Weigel, R.G., Dinges, N., Dyer, R. & Straumfjord, A.A. (1972). Perceived self-disclosure, mental health, and who is liked in group treatment. *Journal of Counseling Psychology*, 19, 47–52.

Weigel, R.G. & Warnath, C.F. (1968). The effects of group therapy on reported self-disclosure. *International Journal of Groups Psychotherapy*, 18, 31–41.

Wexler, D.A. & Rice, L.N. (1974). *Innovations in client-centered therapy.* New York: Wiley.

Wiedemann, P. (1983). Alltags- und therapeutische Kommunikation im Vergleich: Möglichkeiten zur Aufklärung der Therapeut-Klient Beziehung. [Everyday and therapeutic communication compared: Possibilities for clarifying the client-therapist relationship] In D. Zimmer (Ed.), *Die therapeutische Beziehung.* [The therapeutic relationship] Weinheim: Edition Psychologie.

Wilkins, W. (1973). Expectancy of therapeutic gain: An empirical and conceptual critique. *Journal of Consulting and Clinical Psychology*, 40, 69–77.

Wilson, G.T. & Evans, I.M. (1976). Adult behavior therapy and the therapist-client relationship. In C.M. Franks & G.T. Wilson (Eds.), *Advances in behavior therapy.* New York: Brunner/Mazel.

Wilson, G.T. & Evans, I.M. (1977). The therapist–client relationship in behavior therapy. In A.S. Gurman & A.M. Razin (Eds.), *Effective psychotherapy.* Oxford: Pergamon.

Wogan, M. & Norcross, J.C. (1985). *Dimensions of therapeutic skills and techniques.* *Psychotherapy*, **22**, 63–75.

Wolpe, J. (1958). *Psychotherapy by reciprocal inhibition.* Stanford CA: Stanford University Press.

Wolpe, J. & Lazarus, A.A. (1966). *Behavior therapy techniques: A guide to the treatment of neuroses.* New York: Pergamon.

Wrightsman, L.S. & Deaux, K. (1981). *Social Psychology of the Eighties.* Monterey: Brooks/Cole Publishing Company.

Zielke, M. & Kopf-Mehnert, G. (1978). *Der Veränderungsbogen des Erlebens und Verhaltens (VEV): Manual.* [The change questionnaire of experience and behavior (VEV): Manual] Weinheim: Beltz.

Zimmer, D. (Ed.) (1983). *Die therapeutische Beziehung: Konzepte und empirische Befunde zur Therapeut-Klient Beziehung und ihrer Gestaltung.* [The therapeutic relationship: Concepts and empirical findings regarding the therapist-client relationship and its formation] Weinheim: Edition Psychologie.

Index